UNASHAMED

Why do people pay for sex?

A memoir by Elizabeth G.

First paperback edition published in Great Britain September 2024 by
Elizabeth G. Publishing

Copyright © Elizabeth G., 2024

ISBN 9798338847060
Also available as an eBook

Elizabeth G. asserts the moral right to be identified as the author of this work.

All rights reserved. No part of this publication may be reproduced, stored in a retrieval system or transmitted in any form or by any means, electronic, mechanical, photocopying, recording or otherwise, without prior written permission of the author.

While every effort has been made to trace the owners of copyright material reproduced herein, the author would like to apologise for any omissions and will be pleased to incorporate missing acknowledgements in any future editions.

Designed and typeset by Palamedes
Cover design by Alan Conde
Author photograph © Andrew Mason

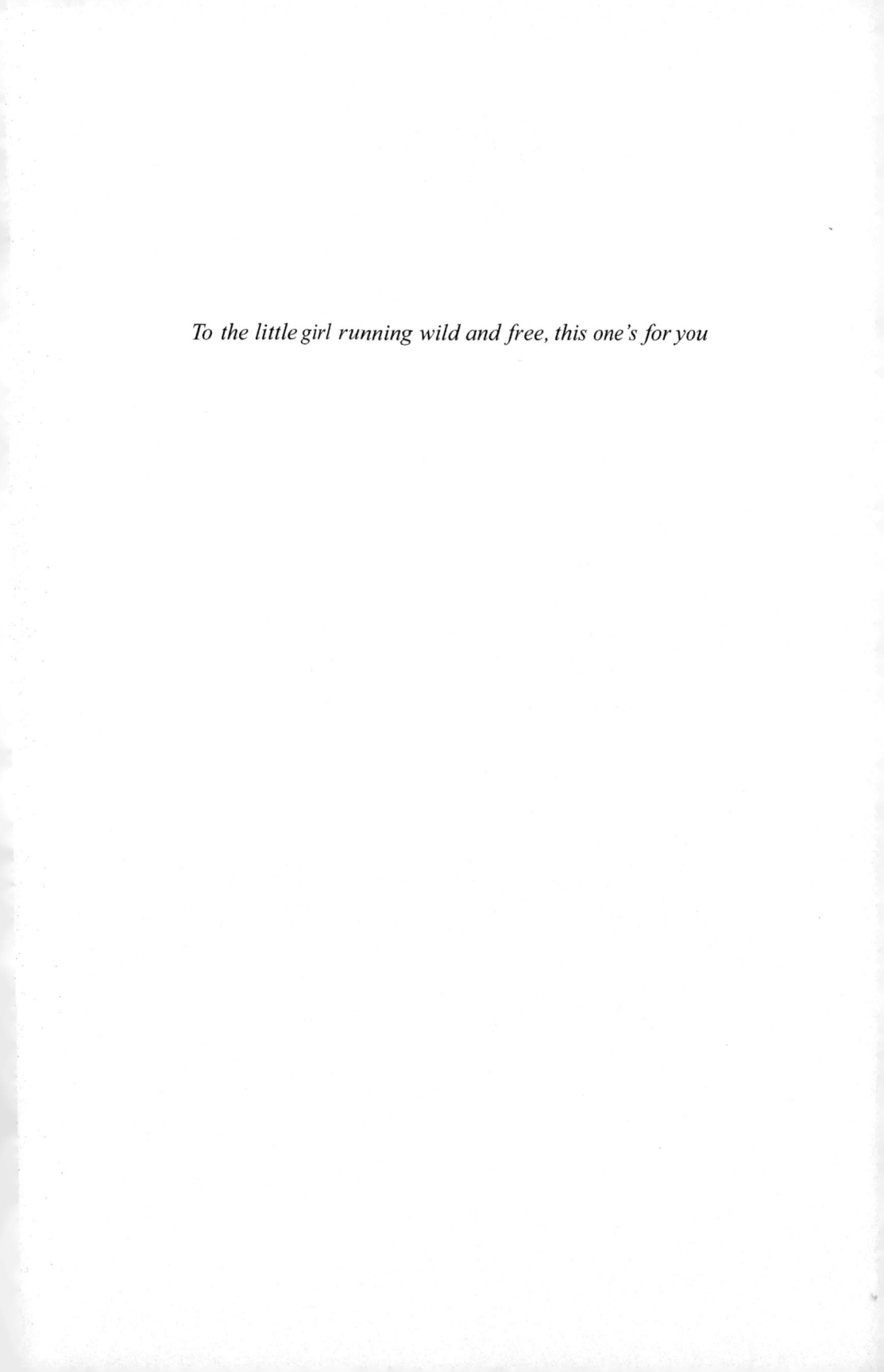

To the little girl running wild and free, this one's for you

CONTENTS

	Prologue	*1*
1.	A Country Girl at Heart	7
2.	First Love	24
3.	Australia	33
4.	Twists and Turns	51
5.	Money Worries	62
6.	Crazy Love	84
7.	Aftermath	108
8.	High-End	125
9.	Momentum	145
10.	Lessons	169
11.	Boundaries	183
12.	Limitless	212
	Epilogue: No More Shame	*224*
	Acknowledgements	*232*
	References	*237*

PROLOGUE

'Why is it immoral to be paid for an act that is perfectly legal if done for free?'
Gloria Allred

It was a beautiful summer's day. The sun was shining, the birds were singing. The background sounds were of glasses clinking, plates clattering, laughter and voices humming while deep in conversation. To anyone looking on, it would simply seem like a happy and relaxed family gathering in the countryside. Conservative and conventional, yes, but warm and friendly too. However, it was social situations like this that would push my anxiety into overdrive.

'How's work going? Have you been busy? Where do you get your clients from? How much do you charge?' I was waiting for the usual questions. Harmless, innocent questions; polite enquiries about my work. But it was exactly these types of questions that I knew I had to try my best to avoid.

As far as my family were aware, I was a massage therapist. This, technically, was true. I had worked as a qualified massage therapist and still very much used that skill as part of my current job. The problem was that I had kept them in the dark as to what that job was. I did not want them to know.

I had to be on my guard. I couldn't socialise like a 'regular' person. Because I had a secret. One that made me feel like there was something wrong with me, like I was a bad person. And I feared my whole family would judge and disown me if they found out. The pressure of keeping that secret made me feel like I had to shut myself off from the rest of the world. It made me live in shame.

ELIZABETH G.

• • •

My first job in the adult industry was when I was a backpacker living in Australia, aged twenty-two. I was short of funds and I heard about a job giving erotic massages with a 'happy ending'. I didn't think too much about it, I just went for it. And I had a blast. I met some amazing women, partied hard and lived the life of a carefree twenty-something with the world at her feet.

I have had other jobs, outside of the adult industry. A lot, actually. I have worked in bars, in property, in marketing. But for many reasons, as you will see, I was continually drawn back to sex work, until, at the time of the pandemic, I was working as a high-end escort in my own apartment in a beautiful area of west London and visiting clients in the city's most exclusive hotels.

A lot has happened since I was that curious young woman, dancing till dawn in Sydney, then travelling up the east coast on the proceeds of the money I made in the erotic massage parlour. My job has allowed me to meet some amazing people, to build a stable financial future for myself and to learn first-hand about the fascinating thing that is human sexuality – including my own.

But some of the lessons I have learnt have been hard ones. I have made mistakes and I have left myself vulnerable to people I can now see it would have been best to avoid. I embarked on toxic relationships with clients, sending me to rock bottom. And, finding myself there, I had to figure out how to get back out again. Compounding – or at the root of – many of the challenging experiences was shame.

From where I stand, I can see that our society views itself as more progressive than it really is. In terms of things like technology, or rights and freedoms for many groups, we have undeniably made progress in the last hundred years. But when it comes to sex, sexuality and sex work, I sometimes wonder if our mindsets have gone into reverse.

Sex, to me, is sensual, passionate, connected, nurturing. Sex has the ability to heal us and bring our senses alive. It's a well-known scientific fact that having an orgasm produces hormones and neurochemicals such as dopamine, which is responsible for feelings of pleasure, desire and motivation. Having an orgasm also increases the number of white blood cells in the body and thus makes it easier for our bodies to fight off infection and potential illness.[1] Having sex is literally good for our brains and bodies. Many papers have been written on the subject. So why is this most natural of human acts still tinged with an enduring hue of shame?

As a sex worker, I see first-hand that we humans crave physical and emotional connection. We are increasingly aware that loneliness is a killer. And yes, there are people who turn to sex workers because they want to explore kinks and fetishes in a space where they don't feel judged. As long as it's consensual and respectful, that's fine with me. But far more visit a sex worker for simple human connection. Because sex workers have the power to heal. A visit to a sex worker, I believe, is all part of a healthy well-being regime. I don't see it any other way.

Sex work is hard graft, though. Yes, it can bring good financial reward. And for many, the flexibility to choose your own hours is a big attraction. But to work as a sex worker, consistently and successfully over a number of years, to build up a good list of regular clients, takes a unique type of person. After all, it's a unique type of job. Sex workers are some of the most misunderstood professionals in the world.

There are many reasons – historical, social, cultural – why we have ended up in this position. Why, when so many taboos have been broken down, sex work still exists largely in the shadows. Just as there are many reasons why someone might decide to be a sex worker or to visit a sex worker. I am not a historian or a sociologist so I won't be unpacking or critiquing those things. This isn't that sort of book.

All I can do is tell you my story. My life as I have lived it. I am very aware of the dark side of the sex industry. When things are pushed underground, demonised, criminalised, there will always be people there ready to exploit that. More precisely: to exploit people. That side of the story has been told and will continue to be told. I fully support that. But that is not my personal experience. My career as a sex worker has been largely positive. My intention is not to encourage, recruit or glamorise my industry. I can't answer for anyone else; I can only speak from my own personal experience.

ELIZABETH G.

In telling my story I have changed names and some locations. I battled shame caused by stigma for many years to get to the place I am in now, where I am writing these words and preparing to tell the truth about my job, to 'out' myself as a sex worker. It's not for me to 'out' anyone else, though.

The sex industry is a multibillion-dollar industry and one of the most lucrative businesses in the world: recession proof, pandemic proof, stock-market-crash proof, extreme-weather proof. In 2009, it was thought that sex work contributed £5.3 billion to the UK economy. Interestingly, it's also the only industry in which women earn more than men. It has been estimated that there are around 105,000 sex workers in the UK.[2] There may be far more. Yet thanks to the stigma and legal grey areas, very little reliable data is available.

Research undertaken by Leeds University and published in 2015, surveying those who identified as having chosen to work in the sex industry, found that 71 per cent had previously worked in health, social care, education, childcare or charities.[3] Thirty-eight per cent held an undergraduate degree and almost all had academic qualifications. In another study from 2015, of 6,570 students, nearly 22 per cent said they had considered sex work.[4] Half of those said this was to pay basic living costs. Nearly half said that curiosity or their own sexual pleasure was a motivating factor.

This industry is not going anywhere. And it will remain appealing to many – especially considering the current economic climate and cost-of-living crisis: soaring mortgage rates, sky-high food prices, huge energy bills, petrol prices. The sex industry is gaining momentum. New online platforms such as OnlyFans add weight to the industry's growth. Let's open our eyes and ears to the reality of that. The more that society buries its head in the sand about sex workers, the more power that gives to sex traffickers, rogue agencies and rogue clients. But the stronger our voices become, the more power we have to protect all of those involved in the industry – sex workers and their clients.

The Madonna–whore complex lives on in the way female sex workers are thought of and written about. It is so much easier to see women as helpless victims or transgressive harlots. Surely we, as a society, should have learnt by now that reducing people to stereotypes and denying the lived experiences of individuals gets us nowhere, and even ruins lives? Many of us are kick-ass business-women who use our bodies and our charm, our wit and intelligence to our advantage. I wasn't forced into sex work. I wanted to be a sex worker. I enjoyed it. It liberated me. I found it more degrading working in an office surrounded by misogynistic vultures where there was a clear difference in pay between men and women.

Let's open up the conversation. Let's at least try to hear each other, to understand each other. We don't have to agree, and that's OK. But it is time to start having more open discussions about sex work. And not just about sex work but attitudes towards women and sex in general. There are still many people out there who struggle to accept that some women not only *enjoy* casual sex, but also enjoy casual sex AND getting paid for it. Yes, that's right. We enjoy it. The majority of us are not victims. We are exactly where we want to be.

Shame is a very unhealthy thing. I should know, I lived with it for long enough. Shame causes a person to exist in isolation and fear. It breeds secrecy and vulnerability. On the most basic level, shame of any kind means you hide who you are from those around you. Shame is dangerous. Shame has the power to silence people.

Writing this book has been very challenging at times. Making the decision to put my story out there has felt like a huge pressure. A weight on my shoulders. But I am doing it because I refuse to continue living my life in shame. I want my story to shine a spotlight on the industry so that sex workers can feel safer and less stigmatised, to do what is in my power to help other sex workers not only survive, but thrive within the industry and use it to their advantage. Let's stop treating sex workers like criminals and give them the respect that they deserve. And the freedom to write down 'sex worker' on their CV and not be discriminated against because of it. My dream is that one day soon, when at a family barbecue, someone asks, 'What do you do?' and receives the reply, 'I am a sex worker,' no one bats an eye.

After many years of shame, I have decided that I want to live my life openly and unapologetically as myself. As a sex worker. I hope that with this book, and in the future, I can help others and change the industry for the better. I am starting that here, now, by telling my story. Loud, proud and unashamed.

There are many versions of sex work out there. This is simply my version.

To all sex workers and anyone dealing with shame, you are not alone. I write my story for you.

CHAPTER ONE
A COUNTRY GIRL AT HEART

When I was a little girl, my parents put a lock on the outside of my bedroom door.

They had awoken too many times to find my bedroom empty, sending them out on a frantic search for their missing three-year-old daughter, who was having the time of her life on yet another wild adventure, oblivious to the total chaos she had caused.

I would often wake just before dawn and begin tuning in to the world around me. While the rest of my family were tucked up in bed sound asleep, I would sneak downstairs into the kitchen. I felt such excitement being up before everyone else. First, my instincts would guide me straight to the fridge. With no parent standing over me telling me what I could and couldn't eat, I would the seize the opportunity and gorge myself on whatever delights caught my eye – leftover potatoes and roast chicken were my favourites. With a belly full of food, I would quietly approach the back door. I knew I had to proceed with caution if I didn't want to get caught. Somehow, I figured out a way to unlock and open the door that towered over me. Out in the countryside pre-dawn, you can almost hear a pin drop. With my parents and my brother still sleeping, it felt like the whole world belonged to me.

There was now just one obstacle remaining: the garden wall. Not for one moment was I deterred. I piled up some leftover bricks one by one, just high enough for me to step onto and make a leap for it. As soon as I was over the wall I was off and running as fast as I could into the distance, stopping at nothing until I got to my digger trucks where I had left them in the mud. In that moment, I was totally free and the world was my oyster. My world being the farm, the natural habitat where I belonged. The possibilities felt endless. I felt like a caged animal being released back into the wild.

Nature and country life were very important to me from an early age. Being raised on a farm was like a having the world's biggest playground on my doorstep – so much room to play, so much space, so much freedom. There were no barriers, no restrictions. I was free to explore and use my imagination. No right, no wrong, no rules. There I was, a joyful, vibrant child who had a thirst for adventure and the great outdoors. I felt free to be whoever and whatever I wanted to be.

Indoors I was restless and energetic. 'You'd destroy a room in seconds. I had the health visitor come to visit. We turned our back and in almost an instant you had gone through all the drawers and pulled everything out. You were just so quick. The health visitor said you'd be very bright,' my mother once told me. So, perhaps it was inevitable that I was always going to live life in the fast lane.

Some of my earliest memories are also some of my happiest. I was bought my first pony, Teddy, when I was around five. This began a lifetime love affair with horses. My mother was a keen horse rider too and was always there to help me with the grooming, feeding and mucking out. We started small with local gymkhana events. In the early years, Mum would run alongside me, one hand on the reins guiding me. Dad was often there too, cheering me on with his great big camera recording all my highs and lows, sometimes with my mother's running commentary heard in the background. From local gymkhanas, we progressed to showjumping, cross country and Pony Club and from there, on to eventing in my late teens.

Back then, Dad recorded pretty much everything, from school plays to Maypole dancing on the village green to trips to the zoo. There are videos of him teaching me to water-ski. It must have taken me about four summers but eventually I got it. No matter the occasion, my parents were always there to support me. They had a very strong presence throughout my early years.

My older brother, Edward, and I never really squabbled. If ever there was a disagreement, I would usually be the one to antagonise him – the stereotypical annoying little sister who walked around like butter wouldn't melt. Sometimes the antagonising came in the form of whacking my brother on the head with the solid metal fire poker, for which he got the blame – 'Edward, stop annoying your sister!' His revenge was telling me there were sweets at the bottom of a sleeping bag and watching me nosedive headfirst, only to find that the sweets were a lie and I was suddenly trapped inside.

The farm under snowfall was heavenly. Dad would bring out his homemade sleighs and my brother and I would spend hours pulling each other around the farm, the dog bouncing around us and playing in the snow. If the snow was deep enough, Dad would bring out his water-skis, attach a rope to the back of the jeep and have someone tow him down the back lane.

My parents grew potatoes on our farm, so potatoes were a common theme for every dinner occasion – a jacket potato accompanied pretty much any meal. Hearty 'meat and two veg' meals were our staple, with the meat coming from my uncle's butcher's shop.

Dad had a cherry tree on the farm that bloomed into the most beautiful pink blossom during the spring and became my tree house, courtesy of my dad's 'handyman extraordinaire' skills. As you might expect from a farmer, my dad was very practical and hands-on. If ever anything needed repairing, drilling, mending, he was there.

When I was nine and Edward sixteen, he left home to go into the army. So from this age onwards, I lived almost like an only child. Nobody to play with or to antagonise. I got used to being around adults pretty much exclusively when I was at home. Still, I was fortunate enough to have my horses, which at that point were my entire life.

During the winter months, my father and uncle would host a shoot at the farm every other weekend – a chance for all the local farmers to get together, have a day out shooting pheasants and hares, and to socialise. One by one, the 4×4s would arrive, filling up the yard, and the volume of chatter would get louder and louder. I observed curiously from the kitchen window. Farmer after farmer with his shotgun, hip flask and trusted gundog by his side, usually in the form of a Labrador or spaniel, itching to get out into the fields. We were always a family of spaniels, cocker spaniels mostly. On the morning of the shoot, while my father prepared himself with his shooting gear, our family spaniel would be going wild with excitement. She knew.

This was a very typical scene I observed as a child growing up and into my teen years. It was all part of farm life. From when I was knee high, I was out there with the men too, in my wellies, winter coat and mop of blonde curly hair. Then, when I was old enough, I adopted the role of 'beater', which entailed walking through the crops in a group with others, literally beating at the crops with a stick and shouting as loud as we could to drive the pheasants out. If you grew up in a town, taking a child out into the fields for a shoot might seem strange or risky. But in the late 1980s in rural Bedfordshire, this was normal. It was what I knew. Even as a small child, I wanted to go out and play in the muddy fields with the farmers. I was never too shy to go out and socialise with the men. I was playful and cheeky, and took great delight in kicking them between the legs. One of my father's friends started calling me 'Jack'. It's almost as if I had to take on that male persona to fit in among the crowd. It really was a man's world. And, on a somewhat subconscious level, I soon figured out how to 'work' a room of men. They didn't intimidate me.

Those winter days out on shoots were my first real taste of socialising with the adults and some of my happiest early memories. I was the youngest and would absorb the adult conversations like a sponge. I just adored to be outside in the elements walking miles across farmland, connecting with nature, dyke jumping, having Brussels sprout fights with my fellow beaters, who were much older than me and already in their late teens. Coming into the warmth of the farmhouse after a long day out in the cold was like being wrapped up in the cosiest duvet. Our dog would be fast asleep in her bed in the conservatory after a busy day of retrieving, the cat motionless in front of the Aga, purring away.

It's fair to say that I was raised in a traditional, old-fashioned environment where the men would work and the women would stay at home cooking in the kitchen, doing household chores and raising the children. My mother was one of the few who did also work as well as look after the house, and me and my brother. So while we were out in the fields all day, my mother stayed home, preparing for the arrival of our empty stomachs.

As day turned to night, my father's friends packed around our dining table, which was fully stocked with port, whisky, wine and snacks. I can still hear the buzz from the conversations flowing around the table. The laughter, the baritone voices, the clinking of glasses and the smell of homemade pastry. My mother busying away in the kitchen while the male energy flowed around the room.

• • •

There's a cliché that children raised on farms get an idea of the birds and the bees from an earlier age – being quite literally surrounded by nature and animals. But I'm not sure this is always true. City kids certainly are exposed to more and grow up faster because of the environment they are in, and having access to more temptations. Plus they may need to be fairly streetwise from a young age. And anyway, I grew up on an arable farm – it's not like my parents were breeding cows and sheep, which you'd think would lead to questions!

On the one hand, I was quite innocent. But I did have a natural curiosity about sex from a young age. At a primary school friend's birthday party, there was a balloon man making various different animals and shapes. He raised one balloon creation to the crowd of excited children and asked, 'And what is this one?' To which I excitedly replied, 'A willy!' My mother cringed with embarrassment.

A friend bought me the explicit version of the Outhere Brothers' 'Boom Boom Boom'. When my mum heard the (highly sexualised) lyrics she was furious and made me return the CD to my friend. I had no idea what the lyrics were talking about. I hadn't given it any thought. But my mum's horror and attempts to restrict what I could have access to only made me want to know more.

My parents were, to an extent, quite prudish – I have no memory of ever being given the classic sex talk. So I definitely thought of it as an area that was taboo, which probably made me even more curious. However, I was also being raised in an environment dominated by males, surrounded by my father's friends, and I'd often catch the tail end of their naughty talk. So perhaps I subconsciously absorbed at a young age that this was a topic for men to talk about, which was out of bounds for women.

But whatever my parents might have been prepared (or not) to discuss with me, it was the early 1990s, and sex was very much a presence on TV and in popular culture. For example, Saturday night was all about *Baywatch*. I was definitely aware that the men who gathered in our house after the shoots were mesmerised by Pamela Anderson as she ran in slow motion across the TV screen in the corner, in a tight, revealing red swimsuit, across a glistening beach, her enormous breasts bouncing up and down. Growing up around a heavy presence of male energy, I became accustomed to hearing men talk about women as objects and the ones to be desired.

As I came into my teen years, boys and drinking were at the forefront of my mind. Aged fifteen and sixteen, getting served alcohol was the biggest hurdle my friends and I faced. And I desperately wanted some to take to the roller disco. But I had a solution. There was never any shortage of alcohol at home, particularly on a winter Saturday after the shoot. Never one to shy away from an opportunity, it didn't take me long to realise that I could smuggle miniatures from my dad's drinks cabinet into my roller skates while he was happily distracted with his friends at the dining table. *These have been there since forever. I'm sure he won't notice if a few go amiss*, I thought. On top of that, there would always be leftover bottles of beer in the greenhouse, where my father and his friends took their lunch break during the shoot.

So, keeping one eye like a hawk on the kitchen door, I would begin to slowly fill up my roller skates with miniatures. If the opportunity was still open, I'd sneak down into the greenhouse, assess the carnage and start collecting whatever unopened beer bottles I could find. And into my bag they went. It felt like such a huge accomplishment, like I was ten steps ahead of the adults.

Growing into my mid-teens, I couldn't wait to be older. I spent a lot of time on my own in my bedroom listening to music, singing to my heart's content. Music was my absolute remedy for the frustrations of teenage life and striving for independence, from Linkin Park's 'Somewhere I Belong' to Britney Spears's 'Stronger'.

I was a real tomboy growing up and that crept into my early teens. Before getting into house and dance music, I went through an indie rock phase. Baggy jeans, hoodies, beads, tiny vest tops and trainers dominated my wardrobe, completed by my bleached blonde hair, washboard stomach and belly button piercing. I lived for Linkin Park. Their songs connected very deeply with my inner teenage angst. I would sing 'Somewhere I Belong' over and over. I felt that, in a sense, they understood me. Blink-182 also had a huge influence on my teen years. I so wanted to be the woman on the front cover of *Enema of the State*. I loved everything about that photo – the cleavage, the red bra, the red lips, the nurse's uniform, the expression on her face as she cheekily pulled a latex glove over her hand with a 'ready for your prostate massage?' kind of look.

I loved the 'fuck you', non-conforming attitude to society that came with the music of bands like Limp Bizkit. I adored Skin from Skunk Anansie. She had her own sense of style that was different from the rest. I was always drawn to those who were different, who broke the mould. Those who owned and embraced their true selves without apology. These bands helped me to rebel against the strict environment in which I was raised. Of course I can see now that my parents were trying to protect me. But I just saw it as them trying to control me.

So, needless to say, the freedom of country life that I had loved so much as a young child wasn't enough as I grew older. I wanted to expand my horizons as far as they would go. I longed for age, wisdom and experience and hated feeling so young and unwise to the ways of the world. I was like a sponge; I just wanted to learn about people, about life, about myself. I wanted independence. I wasn't scared of growing older, I was excited. Gazing out towards the cabbage fields from my bedroom window, I would often dream of a life far away from the farm. A life filled with excitement, glitz, glam and, most importantly, freedom to be myself.

All throughout these rebellious teenage years, from around the age of thirteen to sixteen years old, I kept a diary. The entries are full of references to boys and drinking with my friends. I read them now and laugh at the level of detail I went into, how exhausting my life seemed, going from one boy to another, one social event to another, my emotions like a yoyo as I tried to figure out who I was. It's quite obvious that I was just your typical horny teenager. My friends and I really were all a bunch of boy-mad young girls learning about sex. In popular culture, it's still often teenaged boys who are depicted as being desperate to lose their virginity, obsessed with sex. I think my diary shows that girls can be just as single-minded!

Some examples:

I can't stop thinking about Steven, he's so gorgeous & sexy I just wish I could shag him!

20 January 1997 (aged thirteen)

I had to be in at half past one. So Reese offered to take me home so I said OK. We climbed through the hole in the fence. We seriously started to get off with each other, he fingered me with about 3 fingers and groped me on the tits.

2 March 1997 (aged thirteen)

This Saturday we are all going to Victoria's sleepover in her garden with tents and I'm planning on getting pissed coz I've nicked some vodka out of my Dad's drinks cabinet!

9 July 1997 (aged thirteen)

I LOVE BOBBY ANDERSON. Went with him 13.9.97. He is a bit frigid but quite good looking.

15 September 1997 (aged thirteen)

I had many crushes during my early teenage years. Cobra from *Gladiators* was one (I was fortunate enough to sit on his knee and have my picture taken with him during a signing). Leonardo DiCaprio was another. After watching *The Basketball Diaries*, I was convinced we were destined to be together. Back in the real world, though, my fixation on any one particular person barely lasted five minutes. My attention would constantly flit from one boy to another. One minute I was in love with Steven Anderson (who, to me, was Bedfordshire's version of Leonardo DiCaprio). The next minute I fancied his cousin Bobby. And then, before you knew it, I had a secret crush on my DT (Design Technology) teacher. My diary tells me that I spent one evening playing 'quick fire' blind date in the park with my friend Nadia, choosing Steven and later getting fingered by him at the back of the swimming pool.

My diary also records how, when I was fifteen, my friends from school and I conjured up an ingenious plan. We would congregate at Victoria's house, as she lived only a short distance from town. Her mum and stepdad were away for the evening so the house was all ours. There, we would have pre-drinks before walking into town for a wild night of boys and booze. In order to evade detection from our parents, we would take the phone off the hook (this was before we all had mobile phones) just before leaving the house. So, if any of the parents were to call, the phone would beep as if we were on another call.

One by one we were dropped off by our unsuspecting parents for an innocent sleepover. The night was ours. Giddy with excitement, we began the process of getting ready. Make-up, short skirts, booze in hand and we were all set for our night out on the town, so pleased with ourselves that we had put together the most brilliant plan.

The night became a bit of a blur. Eventually, the group staggered back to Victoria's house, with Nicole (a girl from our group and my usual partner in crime) and I trailing way behind at the back with a couple of boys in tow. We suddenly noticed a commotion ahead of us. We edged slightly closer, still keeping a cautious distance. We suddenly realised that there was a group of angry adults at Victoria's house. Not just any angry adults – angry parents! Our ingenious plan had failed!

'Smack!' Victoria's dad slapped her across her face.

Abort, abort! Horrified at the sight of this, Nicole, the two boys and I started running as fast as we could in the opposite direction, in total fear of the angry parents catching up with us. Luckily, I hadn't seen my own parents there and assumed that they had not swapped contact details with Victoria's parents, so as far as I was concerned, I had got away with this one.

We cut through to the graveyard. In the pitch black I lost one of my Kicker heels, but stopping to find it didn't even cross my mind. The fear of the angry parents catching up with us kept me going.

It was late at night and we had nowhere to go, having told our parents we'd be staying at Victoria's. The original plan of sleeping in our sleeping bags at Victoria's house was officially shot to shit. Plus, I was walking around town with only one shoe. The four of us stuck together looking for somewhere to take shelter for the rest of the night.

For whatever reason, we made our way over to another church and sat down in the archway. The night was cold, we were all freezing. The boys did their best to comfort us and keep us warm – though this amounted to tearing off a couple of pieces of paper off the church door and setting light to them, which lasted all of around thirty seconds. We tried to sleep but it was near impossible.

Once dawn finally started to break, I decided it best to head over to my brother's house in town. With my head held low, I knocked on the door.

'You better come in,' he said with a straight face.

I realised at that point that I was in a whole world of trouble. Back at the farmhouse, I got the third degree. My parents were furious. It turned out that my absence had not gone undetected. My parents had been up all night worried sick about where I was and had had the police out looking for me.

And yet they didn't seem relieved to see me at all. My mum looked like she wanted to kill me: 'Did you sleep with anybody?!!' she said through gritted teeth, bending down and looking me straight in the eyes.

'No,' I said.

I was made to go to the police station with my parents to get a lecture about the effects of drinking and my night of going AWOL. My dad told me that I had a police record for underage drinking – untrue, of course, but his way of scaring me into not drinking. The thought of having a police record did scare me but it wasn't enough to stop me from drinking again. The urge to rebel was too strong.

As an adult looking back on this event, I question how hard the police looked for us or if they even looked at all. In hindsight, we wouldn't have been difficult to find. We were in an open archway to a church only a few streets away from Victoria's house. Not only that but when we were walking around town, I only had one shoe on. If that didn't scream dodgy-looking teenage runaway then I don't know what does.

I had told my mum the truth – I didn't sleep with anyone that night. I think Nicole and I were feeling too scared to get turned on. The boys didn't even try, even though it would have been the perfect opportunity for them. We were vulnerable. They were gentlemen in that sense, even though they were only teenage boys. (Or maybe they were as panicked by the situation as we were.)

Little did Mum know that I had already lost my virginity nearly two years earlier. I didn't think that was the best time to bring it up.

• • •

My first ever 'relationship' was with a boy named Oliver Davies. I was in my final year at primary school, he was the year below me. A 'toyboy'. It was during a school trip to Cornwall that we became 'official'. Holding hands and kissing on the lips felt so exciting, so grown up. Around this time I also enjoyed arm wrestling the boys at school, winning every time. Feeling at ease among the boys at primary school made for a tough transition to an all-female secondary school.

However, I made friends there and it was through my friendship group that I learnt about sex. The only 'conversation' on the subject I remember ever having with my mother was a stern warning not to get myself pregnant. During some of our sleepovers when we had the whole house to ourselves, my school friends and I would go snooping in our parents' bedrooms, often finding their porn collection hidden in the drawers under their bed. This was where the real learning about sex began. That, plus hearing first-hand accounts from those who had already had sex. Watching the VHS tapes we found, we would look on with curiosity, fascinated and giggling at the same time. I was so keen to learn, not just about sex, but about my own body and how it functioned.

One day during Latin class, I decided to start passing a note around that read: 'When giving a blow job, do you blow or suck?' The name suggested you blow, but somehow that didn't make sense in my mind. I needed confirmation from my friends, but nobody seemed to know the answer and the note returned without a response.

Of course, we had the standard 'how to put a condom on a carrot' demonstration at school and a video shoved in front of us. But nobody ever sat me down and explained to me about having sex, about female body parts, about male genitals. Perhaps that was the norm for a child of the eighties.

Losing my virginity came easily to me. I was stone-cold sober. He was twenty-four, I was fourteen. I wasn't taken advantage of. I was consenting. I was curious and keen to lose my virginity and get it out of the way so that I could build on my experiences. Some of my friends in school had already had sex; I wasn't the first in my peer group. I wanted to learn and was ready to experience sex for the first time. He was just a guy I met in a bar; I wasn't in love. I really didn't think that was necessary.

• • •

As a teenager, freedom and independence was always at the forefront of my mind. But thanks to my upbringing on the farm, understanding all the hard work that farming entails, I never expected everything to be served to me on a silver platter. I had been spoilt in a sense with ponies and horses, and for that I was hugely grateful. Competing all over the country in showjumping and eventing was such a passion of mine. I know – and I think I realised at the time – that I had a childhood that some young girls and boys could only dream of. I felt extremely fortunate. However, I never thought these things just came by magic. I was always prepared to put the work in. And, growing up on a farm, it wasn't really a choice anyway.

I always remember my very first 'job' and the seed it sowed in learning about work life and resilience. As a child of around six or seven, I would accompany my parents to sell my father's daffodils by the side of the road in a muddy gateway to one of his fields. There we'd sit, with flasks of hot tea and lunch boxes packed with homemade sandwiches, in the back of my dad's blue trailer, more often than not in the freezing cold and pissing rain. I'd be dressed in my Wellington boots and winter coat buttoned up to the top of my neck to keep out the cold, my mittens on strings attached to my coat so they would not get lost. Waiting patiently for customers to come along, we'd pass the time by playing I Spy. I am grateful my parents took me with them, that they involved me rather than keeping me at home wrapped up in cotton wool. Selling daffodils in the cold and rain with my parents was certainly 'working life lesson' number one.

During school holidays in my teen years, I progressed from daffodil seller to clod picker. This entailed long days standing in front of the potato grader – a conveyor belt for potatoes. As the potatoes bounced pass, I had to pick out any clumps of mud or mouldy-looking potatoes. It was a real family affair; I often worked alongside my older cousin Georgia as well as my dad and my uncle.

'The more you look at it, the slower it will go!' I remember my cousin once shouting over to me as I glanced down at my watch. She was right.

I would often find myself daydreaming to pass the time. Those daydreams took me far away from life on the farm, sometimes to some exotic location by the beach.

Those long days spent potato grading were dusty and noisy. Loud machinery was on the go constantly. It was hardly the glamorous life but something that I grew accustomed to and was grateful for all the same. It was such a buzz to receive the cash in my hand at the end of a long working day.

When I started studying for my A levels, I got a Saturday job working in my uncle's butcher's shop in my hometown. Apart from a brief stint as a waitress, this was my first real experience of customer service and it was terrifying to start with. But once I found my feet, I began to really enjoy this job. The more I began talking to customers, the more my confidence grew.

I had a tin money pot at home. What had previously been a case for a bottle of Malibu was now my 'piggy bank'. After each Saturday shift, I would take my hard-earned cash back home, put it in my money pot and watch it grow week by week. When my savings had reached £100, I felt such a huge sense of accomplishment. It felt good to see my money grow.

Work, to me, symbolised independence and breaking away from the reliance on my parents. Financial independence meant they could no longer dictate to me how to live my life. From a young age, I wanted to work.

As an adult looking back, I feel a deep sense of gratitude for those early career experiences. Especially working on the farm. Farm work was the making of me. Farm work is hard graft. It really is a labour of love. It's physical, it's demanding, it's dirty and totally exhausting. Out in the elements come rain or shine. It taught me tolerance and resilience. It taught me discipline and focus and gave me a new-found appreciation for how hard my dad worked. I am so proud of my country roots and grateful for those early life lessons working on the farm.

I may have begun thinking towards some vague future in which I could have the freedom to go off and have adventures and be whoever I wanted to be. But at that point in my life, the farm, my school, my friends, my parents were all I had ever known. I had no idea that everything was about to change. That my whole world was about to be turned upside down. Aged sixteen, I was about to find out something I had never expected.

• • •

One autumnal Friday afternoon after school, I found myself home alone, doing the usual things that a teenage girl does – looking for food and thinking about boys. My biggest concern that day, as ever, would have been when my next night out would be and what I would wear. I was loitering in the kitchen when I noticed a brown envelope that had been left on the windowsill. It had my first name handwritten on it. Curious. Of course, I took a look inside. As I began to sift through the contents, I noticed that it contained mainly documents relating to my birth. I also saw that there was a letter. I opened it up and began to read:

UNASHAMED

12 January 1984
Dear Mr & Mrs XXXX,

I am writing to give you further information about the baby now placed with you for adoption so that you can keep it for future reference.

Elizabeth was born at XXXX County Hospital on the XXXX at XXXX a.m. Her birth weight was 2730g and it was a normal delivery. Elizabeth has had her full medical examination and this was satisfactory.

Elizabeth's mother, XXXX, is thirteen years of age. She is five feet four inches tall and has dark brown hair, hazel eyes, a creamy complexion and is of average build. She is at present attending Secondary Modern School and doing quite well there. She has a friendly, outgoing but somewhat immature personality. She enjoys horse riding and swimming. Her father is deceased and her mother is a housewife and she has one brother.

Elizabeth's father, XXXX, is eighteen years of age. He is five feet five inches tall, has fair hair, blue eyes and has a tanned complexion and is of average build. He attended Secondary Modern School and is at present working for the Forestry Commission. He is a friendly person but inclined to be irresponsible and enjoys shooting, cars and motorbikes. His father is an engineer and his mother is a hospital orderly and he has three sisters.

XXXX and XXXX met each other at the farm where XXXX keeps her horse. They have known each other for about a year and their friendship is continuing. XXXX has shown interest in her baby and visited her in the foster home. XXXX and XXXX however feel they are too young to offer the baby a happy and secure home and that it would be in her best interests to be placed for adoption.

I also have to let you know that you should tell Elizabeth about her adoption and origins. You should also know that when she attains eighteen years of age (seventeen years in Scotland) she will have the right to obtain a copy of her birth record. A counselling service is now provided for adopted persons should they wish to seek advice on any problems relating to their adoption.

Yours Sincerely
XXXX
Adoptions Officer

The world around me stopped. Total and utter disbelief. I couldn't comprehend what I had just read. My name. My date of birth. My body froze and I went into a state of shock. The hairs on the back of my neck stood on end. I began to have an out-of-body experience; it was as though I was a spectator looking down on myself, taking in this confusing and distressing information. I gazed out of the window, looking out towards the farmyard.

My intuition guided me outside to the stables. I needed the reassurance of the horses. Without really knowing what I was doing, I began mucking out. One motion after another, using the fork and shovel to dispose of the used straw into the wheelbarrow. I was there physically, but mentally I was in a completely different place, almost in a trance-like state. I may as well have been on the moon.

The life I had been living was a lie. All my family had been lying to me. They weren't my biological family, but had pretended that they were. *If this is not my biological family,* I thought, *then who the hell am I? Where is my identity?* As if being sixteen wasn't hard enough, now this bombshell. Life as I knew it was over and in its place, a new life complete with a fresh set of challenges.

I couldn't believe how young my birth mother was. I immediately felt a huge sense of gratitude that she kept me, that she gave me a chance at life rather than having an abortion. Getting pregnant was a big fear among my friends and me at the time. Something we were constantly being warned about. I didn't feel angry with my birth mother, just extremely grateful to have been born. It made me think that I could so easily not have been here. It felt as though I had a new-found appreciation for life. And to say that she had an 'immature personality' was just ridiculous! She was only thirteen years old! Younger than me.

I began to backtrack my whole life up until this point. A lot did start to make sense. Why me and my parents weren't very close. Why I always felt like the black sheep of the family. But never in a million years did I actually think that I was born into another family altogether. It had never even crossed my mind.

All weekend, I kept this piece of life-changing information to myself. A whole weekend of digesting this information on my own, at just sixteen years old. I was scared and confused. And still in a state of shock. That weekend, we went to visit my grandma. It was such a surreal experience. I was looking at her with a completely different set of eyes. My viewpoint had changed. I felt an overwhelming sense of isolation. I began to mentally disconnect from my family. How could they not have told me? My trust in them had all but vanished.

CHAPTER TWO
FIRST LOVE

'Lizzie, you have to talk to your parents about it,' my friend Jessica said.

After keeping my silence for the whole weekend, I had gone straight to her on Monday morning at school and told her everything, showing her the letter.

I knew she was right, but my heart sank at the thought of confronting my parents about it. As hard as it was going to be, it just had to be done. *This is not normal for a sixteen-year-old*, I thought. *This is the sort of thing that adults deal with, not teenagers.* I had spent so much of my teenage years wishing to be older, but I was still a child. This was too much. And for me to be the one to bring it up just seemed wrong. It was my parents' responsibility, but they had chosen to hide it all these years. They had just left the envelope lying around, and now I had seen it. Now I knew.

The next evening, while sitting on the kitchen floor by the Aga, stroking the cat, I looked up to my mum and asked her the question; 'Am I adopted?'

'What makes you think that?' she said, with a surprised look on her face.

'Something I read,' I said, pointing to the envelope.

'You shouldn't read things that don't concern you,' was her reaction.

I was totally bemused. Clearly the letter did concern me.

'We'll talk about this later,' she said abruptly. Looking back, I think she was completely shocked.

And with that, my mother and father were out of the door heading to a meeting. There I was again, left on my own to digest the information with no one but the cat and the dog for comfort.

Later that evening they returned. As I sat on my bed trying to make sense of the situation, my dad came into my room. Looking away from me and out of the window, he very clearly said, 'Well, legally we are your parents.'

I listened. But in that moment I felt like a frightened little girl. I wasn't angry with them, I was in desperate need of a hug, of some love and reassurance. Someone to tell me that everything would be OK, that if I ever needed anything they would be there to listen and to comfort me. But there was just no emotional nurture. It was all so matter-of-fact.

That same evening, my older brother tried his best to help. 'It is strange ...' he said.

It turned out that he had been adopted too, from a different family. My parents told him when he was young, but he didn't take the news well and as a result he had issues in school. He had also known all along that I was adopted, but had never said anything. Because of my brother's reaction, they'd intended to tell me when I turned eighteen. But fate had a different plan.

As an adult looking back, I can clearly see that the way this whole situation was handled was a total mess. It was that lack of comfort, the lack of reassurance, that made it even more unbearable. I began to shut down. I became shy and withdrawn, unsure of who I was, with no sense of identity and a total lack of trust in anyone and everyone. I felt totally disconnected from them all.

The truth is, there is never a perfect time to tell a person that they are adopted. It's always going to be shocking, unsettling, upsetting. What's important is that the child or adult has adequate reassurance, love and nurture surrounding them and is not just left to deal with it on their own like I was. A seed was sown that day.

Still, I had my diary for comfort:

How my feelings have changed! I'm not really sure who I like at the minute but my love life isn't exactly at the top of my list at the minute; my family life is. I

ELIZABETH G.

just want to see what my real parents look like but actually meeting up with them, I'm not so sure about.

20 October 1999 (aged sixteen)

A month later, I was still preoccupied with the same thought:

I really feel that I want to meet up with my natural parents, the curiosity is killing me, and especially as me and Mum are always arguing, like just a minute ago. It's a Saturday night and I've actually stayed in which I deeply regret. I just feel like getting tarted up and going out and getting totally pissed and socialising but I guess I'll have to save it until next weekend.

20 November 1999 (aged sixteen)

I'm not into playing the blame game. Blaming is counterproductive. I take full responsibility for my actions. It's important, however, to acknowledge that whatever kind of childhood you had, it shapes you, and mine absolutely did. Understanding the impact of your family's behaviour is the only way to learn and grow. In recent years, I've learnt to acknowledge the impact those behaviours had on me. My parents are not bad people. They did the best they could, and we have come a long way since this event. I know they love me; they gave me a blissful upbringing on the farm. They just had trouble expressing emotion. Being a natural nurturer, an empath and a lover of hugs, I found it hard to understand and would often find myself feeling hurt and frustrated. But more recently, I've come to accept it and understand my parents with compassion. They had limitations when it came to expressing their emotions. I am OK with that now because I have learnt to nurture myself.

• • •

A few months later, still reeling, I found myself venturing out with my friends for a night out. Our local town was becoming 'uncool', we decided, and so we began to set our sights on what we considered wider, more exciting horizons – albeit another Bedfordshire town only a thirty-minute drive away.

The weekend before, I'd had quite an eventful New Year's Eve out, in which I'd lost my friends and staggered back drunk (naturally – it was a new millennium!) to my brother's house alone, falling over on the way.

Dripping with blood, I somehow made it back but struggled to get into the house, smearing blood all over his white garage. When my friends came to find me, I was a blubbering mess. So with that in mind, I just wanted a fun night out with my friends. No messy drunkenness, no losing each other, just tipsy fun and dancing the night away. Hooking up with boys was not part of my plan.

I couldn't wear a skirt because of the graze on my knee from falling over the weekend before so I wore smart grey trousers, strappy sandals and a black low-cut corset-style top. We began the evening by venturing into various different bars and pubs before heading to the town nightclub, Icon. My friend Gemma and I were chatting at the bar when I noticed a very good-looking guy standing behind her. I tried to point him out but she couldn't see him. Then, before we knew it, the smoking-hot guy's friend started talking to Gemma.

A moment of opportunity. The hot guy came up to me and said, 'Can I talk to you for a sec?'

I was overjoyed and said, as casually as I could, 'Yeah, sure.'

Once we began chatting, we just couldn't stop. We obviously were very attracted to each other and wanted to find out more about each other. His name turned out to be Joshua. He was twenty-three years old and in the RAF. He drove a BMW and a motorbike and also had a dog called Bella. He was originally from Swansea.

We clicked instantly. At first I told him I was eighteen and he believed me, but after we had been talking for a while, I came clean and told him I was sixteen. He didn't seem to mind and told me that he liked younger women – to which I responded by informing him that I was attracted to older men.

We chatted and got to know each other. He asked me for my phone number and I agreed, so off he trotted to find a pen and paper. Soon after, he asked if he could kiss me, to which I happily agreed.

There we were in the middle of the club, connecting in a way that I had never done with the boys I had fancied and messed around with up to that point. All the boys my own age suddenly felt irrelevant. This was new territory – connecting on a deep level with an older man who could not take his eyes off me. They didn't understand me like Joshua did, I decided. I felt noticed and 'seen' in a way that I never had before. It made me feel alive.

He was an incredible kisser, so sensual, and really liked to use his tongue.

'So where would you like me to take you next weekend?' he said very confidently.

He was so forward, but I liked it. He was gorgeous and the age gap was perfect; he was a real man. He showered me with compliments all evening.

We made our way upstairs and found ourselves overlooking the dance floor. I was keeping a close eye on Gemma and the rest of the group. After what had happened on New Year's Eve, I didn't want to lose them.

The time came to around 1.30 a.m. and we had to be leaving.

'You'd better ring me!' I said to Joshua. He promised he would and we said our goodbyes.

Just after 5 p.m. the next day, Joshua called me. I was very pleased to hear from him. He explained that he was reluctant to tell me that he was in the RAF because of the reputation that men in the RAF have. He didn't like the association that they slept around a lot. He told me that he was not into that.

As the days went by, we got to know each other better. He rang me at least once a day, sometimes twice, and whenever he went out, he'd call me on my mobile when he got in, which would usually be around 2 a.m. Even though he'd wake me up, I didn't mind. He always paid me compliments. I started to feel very comfortable talking to him and felt I could tell him anything. I told him about my adoption and he told me that his dad was not his biological dad and how he had adopted him. I had not felt this happy for a long time.

Two weeks after meeting, we got to see each other again. He came to the farm. I had decided that I wanted to start going out with him. He had already told me that he was ready to be in a relationship whenever I was.

The next night we planned to go out again to the same local town where we met. Joshua came to pick me up. My mum insisted that he came inside the house so she could have a chat with him and give him the third degree about keeping me safe and getting me home at a decent hour.

After picking me up, we went back to his room at his RAF base. I was in a building surrounded by men in uniform – every young woman's dream! We made out in his room, then started to get ready for a night out on the town. We ended up back in the club where we had first met. His friends were out with us too, including the one who'd hit on my friend Gemma, who, it turned out, was married. *What a dick*, I thought.

In spite of that, it turned out to be one of the best nights of my life. I was so happy to be with three older men who were buying me drinks all night and my gorgeous new boyfriend Joshua, who was paying me lots of compliments and waiting on me hand and foot. *I could get used to this!*

As the night progressed and the drinks flowed, I found myself getting more and more drunk. I told Joshua that I loved him and that I wanted to have sex with him. He told me that he didn't love me yet. I felt hurt and frustrated by his response.

Even so, the next minute, we were outside looking for a place to have sex. We went behind the back of a building. I took a condom out of his pocket and began opening it. He stopped me and told me that he couldn't have sex with me because I was too drunk and I would probably regret it the next day. As frustrated as I was, I was at least mature enough to realise it showed he cared about me and didn't just want to use me for sex.

Joshua's friend dropped me off at home in a prearranged 'designated driver' deal. Dad had locked the door so I had to ring the doorbell to get in. It woke my mum up and she came downstairs to let me in. Surprisingly, though, she didn't seem to mind.

At that point in my life, Joshua was everything I could have dreamt of. It's almost as if he was too good to be true. A real gentleman.

Shortly after our amazing night together, Joshua had to go back home to Swansea. While he was away, I had a night out with my friends. One of the girls in the group came up with the most ridiculous game of seeing who could snog the most guys. The winner would be bought a bag of chips.

After drinking more and more, I began to participate in the game, going from one boy to another. I didn't feel guilty. It was just a silly game and the kisses didn't mean anything.

However, when I got home that night, the guilt began to creep in. The following Monday, I decided to call Joshua and come clean. One of the boys in sixth form was giving me a hard time about it, which didn't help, so I thought it better to be honest and open about it. He didn't take the news all that well. He said that he felt gutted and pissed off but at the same time he appreciated my honesty.

After that, things just weren't the same. He didn't compliment me as much and the tone of our conversations had changed. He kept going on and on about some worries he had at work. Valentine's Day was looming but he didn't mention it and I had to remind him when it was. My first Valentine's Day with a real boyfriend who was a grown-up man and he didn't seem to be into it!

One Saturday afternoon, I saw I had a missed call on my mobile. As usual it was Joshua. I called him straight back. He said that he had a 'confession to make'. At first, I thought he was calling me to tell me he had been with someone else behind my back but it was worse than that. He told me he was being posted away next month. My heart sank. It turned out that he had known about this from the moment we met. I was distraught. He had led me to believe that we'd be together for a long time and even said that he wanted me to go with him to Swansea to meet his family and friends. He said that he'd been feeling guilty about it and couldn't lead me on anymore.

It was all so sudden. I was meant to be going over to see him that night. I had been looking forward to it all week. Now I was never going to see him again?

'If you come round tonight, we'll probably end up having sex,' he said.

Well, that didn't bother me in the slightest! I told him that it was better I came over and we had sex rather than not at all. But it was the usual response from Joshua as he began to reiterate that he just wasn't into that.

I began to feel my nose running and my eyes welling up. I was determined not to cry but after I put the phone down I burst into tears. The pain from this news was beginning to burn. It was a level of deep emotional pain I had not felt before. Something about it felt unbearable. I wanted to shut myself away from the rest of the world.

Being a teenager, I quickly changed my mind. I decided that I wanted to go out that night. My parents had plans and were going out. No way was I staying home alone after breaking up with Joshua. I called around all my friends but they were all staying in.

It got to around 6 p.m. I caved and called Joshua. I asked him if he wanted to come over so that we could have a chance to say goodbye. The thought of never seeing him again was so painful. He was my first love and I really didn't want to let him go. But there was nothing that I could do about it. It hurt me so much.

Eventually, after much persuasion on my part, Joshua did come over that evening. It was weird seeing him. I wanted him to stay as long as possible and I didn't care if it made things worse – as far as I was concerned, things couldn't get any worse. We sat in his car before he left and he gave me a hug. 'I'm so sorry,' he said. 'Yeah, so am I,' I replied.

It hurt for a long time, in that uniquely raw way you feel pain as a teenager when everything is new and you have never been let down in love before. I slowly started to get over him – while still daydreaming about going to Swansea University when I turned eighteen and getting back together with him. It wasn't long before I started getting back into the swing of going out with my friends again, returning to the neighbouring town and snogging boys on the dance floor.

Then one Sunday evening, Joshua rang me.

What followed were numerous occasions when one of us would get drunk and call the other. One night when he'd been out in Swansea and was very drunk he kept saying that he wanted to have sex with me the following weekend. I didn't believe him at first, but he kept going on and on about it so eventually, like a fool, I fell for it. I said that if he was serious then he would call me tomorrow and tell me then. He rang the next day but confessed that he'd only said it because he was drunk and didn't really mean it. I was so upset; I'd really got my hopes up, but it was all just alcohol-fuelled.

I can see now that in the period of my life when I met Joshua, I was going through a hell of a lot of teenage angst. Many first romantic relationships are intense, but I think this was especially so considering what had just happened in my life. I met Joshua only a few months after finding out I was adopted. He made me feel safe and secure. So when it all came to an abrupt end and he went back to Wales, it was as if I was reliving the feelings of abandonment from my birth mother all over again.

It became increasingly obvious that there wasn't going to be some heart-stopping Hollywood reunion between us. In fact, it all started to get quite tiresome. At that point, I decided that the best thing to do would be to just let him go even though I still missed him. I knew that I had to forget about him and just get on with my life.

And get on with my life I did.

CHAPTER THREE

AUSTRALIA

Tired and exhausted, I dragged myself home from the bar to the hostel where I was staying, feet throbbing and swollen from an excruciating seven-hour shift. It had been another long night of dealing with rude customers, who became progressively more obnoxious the drunker they got. I couldn't wait to get back to the hostel, de-robe from my beer-sodden uniform and cleanse the night off with a steaming-hot shower.

Fortunately, though, my time working at the bar was coming to an end. The terms of my visa limited me to taking a job for just three months before I had to move on. I was looking forward to never having to set foot behind that bar ever again but, at the same time, dreading having to find another job. Funds were running seriously low.

The November of 2005, after I had graduated from university with a BA in business management and marketing, I left the dark nights and damp days of the British winter to spread my wings and experience life in a different country. There was no way I was going straight from four years of study into a corporate job. I had zero plans, I just couldn't wait to be on the other side of the world, in a whole new place, meeting different people, far away from my family and everything I knew. I craved the space and freedom to be myself.

The only problem was money. At twenty-two, I may have been full of the joys of a wide new horizon, but I was shit at budgeting. I had never been taught anything about money or how best to invest and grow it. When I finally broke free from the boozy chaos of the bar where I was working, my plan was to follow the well-trodden backpacker route up Australia's east coast. Cairns, Airlie Beach, Byron Bay ... I imagined parties on sandy beaches, snorkelling on the reef, maybe meeting some hot boys to share my adventures. But as I made my way home, late at night in the midst of the sizzling Sydney summer heat, I was again worrying about how I was going to pay for it. And, more pressingly, how I was going to fund food and accommodation for the next few weeks.

On the one hand, I loved being in Australia. But it was already tainted by my constant worry about finances. It was eating away at me and made my stomach churn. It felt scary to be so far away from home and fast running out of cash. Even working six days a week at the bar wasn't enough. Going back home to the UK was not an option, though. My new-found freedom meant too much and there was absolutely no way I was going to give that up. Here, I could be whoever I wanted to be.

I could, theoretically, have asked my parents for money, if I'd had to. But I wanted to avoid that at all costs. I was sure it would come back to bite me on the arse somehow. Plus it made me feel guilty just thinking about it. To be truly free in this exciting new place I had to manage somehow. I had to rely on myself.

I let myself into the hostel.

About a thirty-second walk to the beach and across the road from the bar where I worked, the hostel was located on a side street overlooking a cricket ground. It was an ideal location for any backpacker. I was sharing a room with two other female travellers. We had our own kitchenette and bathroom so it was a step up from sharing amenities with a whole building of other travellers. I'd get in at different times depending on my shift, which would most typically be from around 5 p.m. to midnight. More often than not, my roomies would be out by the time I got home, giving me a chance to unwind after a long night. If they were around we'd either meet for a Garlo's pie on the beach or, if we were in the mood for something a bit livelier, we'd get changed and go off into the night to dance the night away among the bright lights of Sydney's Kings Cross. (Which partly explains where all my money was going.) My hours at the bar meant that I'd have all day to recover. It was not uncommon to party with work colleagues too. Despite not liking the job itself, I worked with a great bunch of people. One evening, one of the hot Australians I worked with made a move on me and we ended up having sex in the rock pool by Coogee Beach. Working in the bar did have its perks!

As I cleansed off the evening and changed into my pyjamas, my mind slowly began to untangle from my financial woes. It was as though my intuition was guiding me and reassuring me that everything would be OK. Once my body began to feel at ease, I fell into an exhausted sleep.

• • •

A few days later, I was in the pub with my friend Sasha. We got talking about work and finances. She was there with her friends Lucas and Andre, who were a couple. I was drawn to Sasha as soon as I met her; she had a real vibrancy about her. She was similar in age to me and a total hedonist too. We both had a love for partying and shared the same taste in music, from dance, electronic and indie to the Doors, Faithless and the Prodigy. Sasha was very down to earth and easy to talk to – I felt comfortable around her. She was just as excited to be exploring Australia as I was. She was beautiful and had a great sense of style; she wasn't afraid to be unique and stand out. I looked up to her.

She had a new job, but it took a while to get to the bottom of what it actually was. It was in Sydney's Inner West. It wasn't waitressing. She would begin telling us but then break off, giggling, as if unsure of how we would react. Eventually, she came out with it – she was working in an erotic massage parlour, performing naked massages on male clients, with a 'happy ending'.

The boys hooted with laughter, enthusiastically showing their support for Sasha's new job. 'Go for it, babe! I would absolutely do that if they would let me! Wait, would they let me?' said Lucas, as his boyfriend playfully punched his arm. I was intrigued. Actually, more than intrigued – I was fascinated.

I knew very little about the sex industry at the time, but it had always interested me. When we were in sixth form, a school friend had seen an advertisement in a lingerie shop in town looking for models and asked if I wanted to join her in applying. Pat, who we quickly nicknamed 'Pat the pervert', claimed his photographer was from *FHM*. We were suspicious but enticed by the promise of glamour modelling success. Of all the 'lad mags' of the nineties and noughties, *FHM* was top of the pile. Their annual '100 Sexiest Women in the World' poll and 'High Street Honeys' – for which women around the country sent in photos of themselves – helped define what we thought of as sexy. Or what we thought boys thought was sexy. Which to us then was the same thing. So I did not hesitate – any chance of getting into the magazine was worth it.

My friend and I went along to the location we were given, which turned out – slightly bizarrely – to be next to a local garden centre just outside of town. The photos, for reasons I cannot fathom, were taken inside a greenhouse. Was it warmer? Are greenhouses sexy? Our make-up was done by a lady who made me look like her very own amateur drag queen creation. I had purple eyeshadow painted on up to my eyebrows. Some shots were taken of me in my underwear and some in a camouflage jumpsuit complete with a fake wooden gun and heels. Shortly after the 'photoshoot' we were given copies of the photos. I made sure that they were tucked away safely in the deepest, darkest corner of my bedroom and kept far away from the detection of my parents. We were not called up by *FHM*, pleading with us to be their next cover stars. I don't know what became of the pictures, but it didn't really bother me.

Later, when I was at university, I also applied to work in a strip club – despite having never actually been in one. Getting well paid (in my student eyes) to dance around in little to nothing seemed like a good deal to me. Though not only was I turned down by the club, but my mum read my email. There was no discussion about it. She just said one word: 'DON'T!' And we left it at that.

I think what really grabbed my interest was the lifestyle, the glamour, the partying. The minimum effort for maximum profit. The idea that you could get paid for being an object of desire was incredibly alluring. At the time, to be desired felt like the biggest achievement and compliment. Don't forget that the late nineties/early noughties was the era of the glamour model. Katie Price (or Jordan, as she still was), Melinda Messenger, Carmen Electra. These women, to me, appeared to have it all; the house, the holidays, the cars, financial independence and men lusting after them.

Also, I was very much a free spirit, just as I am today. The sex industry enticed me because there didn't seem to be a set routine and there appeared to be more freedom to work and also play. I think it's also worth noting that I was very much of the rebellious, non-conforming type. I never dreamt of getting married and having children. The thought of living a 'regular' life in an office or being a stay-at-home mum with 2.4 children living down a cul-de-sac terrified me. I craved excitement. I wanted to live my life differently. My parents put such an expectation on me to get a degree and get a 'good job' in an office. But I hated the idea of living a monotonous routine. I felt like it would be the equivalent of being brain dead. (Later I was to find out that working in an office did make me feel exactly that – like a total zombie, and deeply unhappy. It's just not for me.)

So when I heard about my friend's new job it seemed like a great opportunity to find out more about the sex industry, something I'd always been interested in. I was confident in my body and being desired felt like the ultimate goal. I knew I could do this. And then I heard how much my friend was making – around $3,000 a week. To socialise, party, sit in hot tubs drinking champagne, wank off a few guys?! I had dollar signs in my eyes and began to fantasise about what I could do with that amount of cash, about all the travelling I could do. It was the obvious solution to my money worries. I was sold.

The application process was very straightforward: I just had to send them a few photos, have a chat on the phone and Sasha would put in a good word for me. The receptionist seemed very friendly and invited me in for a trial.

On my very first day at Tantra House, I got the bus from Coogee Beach, taking me from the Eastern Suburbs through to Bondi Junction and on to the Inner West of Sydney. It was like I was in a trance for the journey, in some kind of zone mentally preparing myself. I was excited but incredibly nervous. I turned to my music to help calm my nerves, playing the same song over and over again on my iPod – 'Alright' by Red Carpet. Almost twenty years later, that song still has the same effect on me – calming, reassuring, but at the same time giving me energy, making me want to get up and dance all night. That song would later be known as 'the Lizzie song' among my friends. Every time we were out at a club or festival, they knew the effect that song would have on me. I just wouldn't be able to stop myself from hugging and holding my friends, telling them how much I loved them.

Upon arrival at Tantra House, I was introduced to the reception team, given a locker and then taken on a tour with one of the other ladies. My eyes must have been out on stalks as I looked around, taking it all in. Tantra House had three floors. The ground floor was the reception and lounge area, with a bar and pool table. The first floor was accessed by a rather imposing spiral staircase and had private massage rooms, communal hot tubs and changing rooms. The lower-ground floor consisted of private suites, complete with a massage table, hot tub and shower. I would soon learn that bookings in the suites were preferable – they were longer, including time spent sitting in the hot tub drinking and chatting, which meant more money.

I had never been in a place like this before. It was a whole new world to me but at the same time I felt like it was where I belonged. I could feel the energy of the rooms. All past experiences in these rooms were whispering to me, enticing me in. I was curious, nervous, excited, intrigued. A whole mix of emotions. It was all so new and surreal but at the same time, I couldn't wait to have experiences there.

The woman showing me around was a local lady in her forties. She seemed friendly enough but didn't go out of her way to make me feel at home. I got the impression that she had done the tour with the 'new person' many times before. She showed me how to fold and roll the towels. It was all very particular. I was told that she was going to do a demonstration massage on me; I was really looking forward to it but don't recall her ever doing that. It was more like, 'Here are the oils, here are the towels, here's how to set up the room,' etc. All the practicalities of the job.

Once a client checked in and entered the lounge area, we were expected to walk up and introduce ourselves one by one, dressed in a most tempting mini skirt, top and heels, or a figure-hugging dress. For clients who wanted to be more discreet, there was a private room where they could wait and meet the ladies. Once we had all introduced ourselves, the receptionist would then ask the client who he'd like to book, what kind of room he'd like and how long for.

I chose Natalie as my work name – we all chose our names for various different reasons. Some ladies who I became close with would tell me their personal name. It's an absolute rookie error to give a real name to a client (and I know this because as a rookie, it's something I did numerous times while under the influence). It felt very exciting to get picked and have my name called out: 'Natalie, you have a booking!' Being 'the chosen one' felt super special, especially in those early days when everything was so new and exciting.

My first client was just a regular-looking guy, the 'geek chic' type – middle aged, glasses, an everyday person you might walk past on the street. I don't think I'd ever felt so nervous as I waited outside the room for him to get ready, but that still didn't stop me. I entered the massage room and he was lying face down on the massage table – naked, of course, as was I. I reached for the oil, which had been kept nice and warm in the heated cabinet, and began massaging it into his back and shoulders. It might sound strange, but I was more worried about the fact that I had absolutely no clue how to give a massage rather than the fact that I was totally naked with a complete stranger and about to wank him off! I asked him to roll over onto his back. As I began to massage his groin area with my back to him, he slipped his fingers inside of me. 'You taste good,' he gleefully told me, licking his fingers. 'Thank you,' I said smiling nervously. It was a natural progression to the 'happy ending'. The client came very quickly and it felt like no effort at all. The booking was over before I knew it. I couldn't believe how easy it was. After the 'nervous first' one was out of the way, that was it. There was no stopping me. I began to fly.

• • •

Tantra House soon became a place where I felt I really belonged. A place where I could have fun, meet like-minded men and women, be free to express my *true* self and get paid very handsomely for it. I soon began to make friends. Some ladies were locals, some were fellow travellers, others were students and single mothers. Tantra House had an array of ladies on offer. Someone for everyone; ladies to suit all tastes. Natural curves, petite, athletic, silicone; blonde, brunette, redheads; British, Australian,

American, Scandinavian, Indian, Thai, Malaysian. Ladies in their twenties, thirties and forties. A bevvy of beauties.

We all seemed to be in tune with each other, perhaps due to a shared understanding of why we were working in the industry. I soon began to learn that sex workers are very sociable and friendly people, naturally caring and good listeners. Some people have an idea of men who visit sex workers as perverts, people you'd cross the street to avoid. But when you do a job like this you realise it is almost like a form of therapy. It is a 'feel good' service after all, and the vast majority of sex workers genuinely want their clients to feel good.

I don't think I thought too deeply about it at the time – I was twenty-two years old, having fun and making money. But I know now that it takes a certain type of person to do this job: a person who has mental strength, confidence and great social skills. A person who enjoys life, is a natural performer, likes to have fun and doesn't take themselves too seriously. So many sex workers I have met are kind and natural healers as well as being business savvy. Obviously being sexually open and free is an important aspect, and of course the money is a big draw, but sex work is so much more than that. Sex work is all about *connection*. The best sex workers are very self-aware and in tune with others. They are very giving and want their clients to leave with a big smile on their face. This was what these women at Tantra House had in common, and it was a big part of the reason why it was so easy to bond with them.

One evening, as I was finishing my shift, I was walking upstairs to the changing rooms when I heard a voice say, 'Oh my God, I love this song!' The volume was cranked up and I began to hear 'Mystify' by INXS blaring out of the speakers. As I walked through the changing room door, a stark-naked blonde bombshell began dancing. 'My kind of woman!' I thought. Her name was Katie, and she was from New York. She would become a very important part of my life and my time in Australia, and on that first meeting, her energy, her zest for life, her sensuality was just so fascinating to me. We clicked instantly.

I was also totally mesmerised by Imogen, a gorgeous Australian in her twenties. A natural beauty, she was petite and curvaceous. Her eyes were intoxicating. She was always as cool as a cucumber and took everything in her stride. She was a student and working at Tantra House to fund her studies. In between bookings, she would often sit at the back of the lounge area with her head in her books. Her parents knew about her working in erotic massage and were supportive. I felt so envious that she had such open and understanding parents who she could talk to about anything.

I also got on really well with Ivy. She was a natural 'glamour-puss' who sported an immaculate manicure at all times. Originally from New Zealand, she was in her forties, a single mother with a grown-up son who she was supporting. She was always very fearful of him finding out about her job. Still, she knew how to have a good time and was a total natural. She had an ability to turn on the charm at the flick of a switch. I watched how she had a very subtle but apparently natural way with clients. She was very attentive and I could see that they always felt like she was really listening to them. I learnt a lot from the ladies at Tantra House, but particularly Ivy. The other important thing I noticed was that she always seemed to be genuinely enjoying herself, something that I have observed over the years and understood to be an essential part of the profession.

Sophie was beautiful and demure. She had a killer smile and was very easy to talk to as well as soothing to be around. We became good friends. One day after working the day shift together, we decided to go to a strip club and pop my 'strip club cherry'. We must have been the only female spectators in the whole venue.

Alicia was really fun to work with. Another blonde bombshell with great energy. She always seemed up for a good time and absolutely oozed sex appeal. She was also an Aussie in her twenties and worked in finance during the day. Unfortunately, she had to leave very suddenly when one of her clients from her corporate job walked into Tantra House.

One thing was for sure: we all knew how to have fun.

Whenever a bunch of super-sexy clients walked into the building, the ladies would be swarming all over them like bees around a honey pot. On the other end of that spectrum, if Alan (one of the venue's oldest regulars) came in, we'd be hiding at the back of the lounge hoping our absence went unnoticed. The receptionist would have to walk over and remind us to be friendly and to go over and introduce ourselves.

Some clients who walked into our lounge would just get a 'Hi, I'm Natalie, nice to meet you.' But if the chemistry felt right and we had a good rapport, I'd sit and chat some more, turn on the charm, ask about their day and get to know them better in the hope they would pick me. Smoking-hot clients were a bonus, but not essential.

An average shift was usually about three to five bookings a night, although this depended on the length and type of each booking. Group bookings in the hot tubs with other ladies were fun and could last hours. We'd drink champagne and listen to music, straddling the jets and laughing our heads off. But I also loved being in the private rooms with a client one on one.

Over time, I began to build up my regulars. Building up regulars was like finding little nuggets of gold. When it was less busy, you could always rely on a regular client walking through the door.

Bookings with them felt like such incredibly easy money. To have fun and party with people that I was genuinely attracted to and got on well with was great – to get paid for it on top of that was just the icing on the cake. We were paid cash and I was definitely earning more than enough – even more than I had hoped. Going home with a wad of cash after each shift was such a reassuring feeling.

As far as my parents were aware, I had been able to extend my time working at the bar. They didn't need to know any further details. They wouldn't have understood. Back then, with no smartphones, no social media, no selfies, no tagging locations for all to see, it was much easier to be elusive. There was a lot more freedom to live our lives without all and sundry knowing what we were doing and when. It was totally freeing.

I was meeting such interesting people, from priests to accountants, builders to company directors, musicians to actors. I just loved to meet people from all walks of life and hear about their experiences of the world. For the most part, it was simply erotic massage with a happy ending. The general rule at Tantra House was not to have sex with the clients, but there were lots of rumours of other ladies giving a 'full service' and I think a blind eye was mostly turned by the management if people were discreet. I had sex with clients on a few occasions in the building – when I was drunk or high and genuinely attracted to them I just thought, *What the hell?* and went for it. I don't remember charging extra. I was just having a great time.

I never had any issues in terms of safety. Of course, the venue was open all hours of the night and into the early morning so there was the odd incident with rowdy drunk clients, though I didn't personally experience any problems. I'm pretty sure the building had cameras but I just didn't really think about it. It was a great atmosphere created by a bunch of amazing women and clients who were happy to be receiving their services.

Early one morning after finishing work, I was waiting outside Tantra House on the opposite side of the road, looking for a cab, when a police officer pulled up in front of me. 'Would you like a lift? It's not safe here.' I accepted his offer and got in. I never felt that Tantra House was in an unsafe area. It was very much in the hipster part of town, full of foodies and farmers' markets during the day and bustling restaurants and bars by night. I thought it was perfectly OK and never had any issues. I think the police officer just fancied giving me a lift home. I'm sure he knew where I'd been all night. It must have been quite obvious. He was smoulderingly handsome. I was always a sucker for a man in uniform and there was just something about the Aussie police. Unlike our PC Plods back in the UK, the Australian police were totally ripped with shoulders to die for (shoulders very much being 'my thing'!).

'So where have you been this evening?' he said curiously.

'Just out with friends,' I said, smiling innocently. I had learnt to use my look of innocence as my greatest weapon. Playing the 'dumb blonde' worked like a charm. Those who have underestimated me over the years have soon realised their mistake. He dropped me home; I thanked him for the kind gesture and we said our goodbyes. I always regretted not asking for his phone number.

Tantra House had very quickly become my world. It wasn't just a job, it was my social life, where I made friends and met men. Not having to worry about money and being free to express myself sexually felt totally liberating. The only downside of the work was feeling the need to keep what I did secret from people outside of that world, for fear of judgement. It was easier to be around people who knew about my job rather than have to deal with the anxiety of hanging around a group that didn't know, waiting for that question, 'So, what do you do?'

Inevitably, I was going to fall for some clients. Because the job is so intimate and is all about building a connection, in the early days at least, when I was young, having the time of my life and new to this world, it was only a matter of time before I'd start to see clients outside of work and even date some of them. It felt like a natural progression.

One of my regulars was from Chicago. He worked in marketing and was an average-looking guy. Suited and booted. He booked me many times and we'd spend hours chatting. I had so much fun getting to know him and I felt really comfortable with him. He absolutely adored me and would hang on my every word. One evening after work, he waited for me in the park opposite Tantra House. Bleary-eyed and still feeling ravenous for each other, we tucked ourselves discreetly behind a tree and began fucking like animals. Having sex doggy style out in the open air with my knickers around my ankles while hugging a tree felt hugely exciting. From there, we went on to his office in the city. While he had me bent over his desk, I caught a glimpse of my reflection in the window. In that moment I thought to myself, *I love my life!* The element of risk heightened my senses and excited me even more.

Another time, we somehow ended up spending the night together in a hotel room. He had to leave early for work in the morning. When I handed the keys in at reception on my way out, the receptionist asked me to confirm the guest's surname. I had no clue. It became very clear to the receptionist that we did not know each other on a personal level. I cringed with embarrassment. The judgement from her eyes felt like lasers burning into me.

Another of my regulars was a builder from the UK. The sexual chemistry between us was insane and I always looked forward to bookings with him; they were guaranteed to be fun and sexy. He'd bring drugs with him and book a private suite. More often than not, he'd extend the booking, which always felt like such a huge win. My ideal was always to spend all night with a client that I connected well with. Sometimes other ladies would join us for some threesome naughtiness.

Just like with the Chicago marketing guy, we ended up expanding our fun times together to outside of Tantra House. We shared a love for partying in Sydney. We'd go out, dance the night away, do drugs together and then go back to his for the afterparty and spend the night fucking the crap out of each other. Admittedly, I was starting to fall for him. While on the one hand this was a bit of a rookie error on my part, it's more common than you might think for sex workers to date clients. I have known many friends to date clients over the years; sometimes it works out and sometimes it doesn't. I know of only one who got married to a client and had children with them. As far as I am aware, the relationship lasted.

For one thing, dating a client takes away the fear factor of having to reveal your job to a guy who doesn't know about it. I am much better at compartmentalising now and I know my boundaries and how important it is to stick to them. But in the early days, when I was a backpacker working at Tantra House, the lines were very blurred. A lot of this was down to the drugs and alcohol. Especially the alcohol. Being drunk with clients, I gave far too much information about my private life away (real name, where I was from, etc.) – many of the ladies did. But now I know better.

There was a big drug culture in Sydney, and being the young hedonist that I was, I embraced it with every ounce of my being. I had been partying and using drugs long before I began working in the sex industry. During my university years, I often visited one of my school friends at Bristol University. It was there that we began going to clubs and taking pills, ecstasy mostly. A trip to Ibiza during this time only confirmed my love for partying and being on the dance floor until sunrise. I was a true raver of the early 2000s. I'd loved dance music from my early teens and would eat, sleep and drink music. For me, taking ecstasy only heightened that feeling. It was the love drug, after all, and always encouraged me to embrace my friends and tell them how much I loved them. If it wasn't my friends, it would be a total stranger that I'd be sitting next to, talking rubbish to all night while massaging their hand! That was the beauty of ecstasy, it was the 'togetherness' drug.

I remember the first time I tried speed. It was during a group booking in the communal hot tub. I watched the client sprinkle some into my drink. As I took one small sip after another, I slowly felt my whole body begin to melt among the bubbles. It was a heavenly feeling and only encouraged my desire to experiment with drugs further.

• • •

I had been working at Tantra House for about two months when a very attractive man named Lorenzo booked me. He was tall, dark and handsome. Great shoulders too, of course! As I entered the massage room, he said, 'You have a beautiful body.' I was very attracted to him and felt incredibly nervous around him. His compliments made me blush. We talked and talked and did not stop. Our connection was obvious from the very beginning. I was surprised that he didn't want the happy ending, just to chat and have a regular massage – maybe that's what lured me in. At the end of the booking, we exchanged phone numbers.

I was on my way home in the taxi after my shift when Lorenzo messaged me. I was so happy to hear from him. I had not felt such a deep connection with a man for some time and it excited me. He continued to shower me with compliments and wanted to arrange meeting up. I happily said yes.

As Lorenzo and I began dating each other, I became totally smitten. He told me he was in a band and played me some of his music. Obviously he knew about my job, so I didn't have to feel bad about hiding it from him or worry about how I was going to tell him. It was all out in the open from the very beginning and he accepted me for who I was. On top of all that, the sex was just incredible. He had Italian blood running through his veins and boy did I know it! Such passion, such charm. I quickly fell for him.

One evening, Lorenzo and I went to the pub to meet some of his friends before I started my shift. It was nice to meet some of his social group and get to know more about him. But then as Lorenzo and I began making our move to leave, one of his friends shouted across the table, 'Where are you guys going?' It was clearly a loaded question. She was almost taunting us. My body froze and I began to feel an internal panic. We hadn't prepared for such a situation. Lorenzo shrugged it off and made something up on the spot, but it didn't sound convincing and I was sure that I had a look of horror on my face. I wanted the ground to open up and swallow me whole. 'But where are you guys really going?' Lorenzo's 'friend' continued the taunting as we made a swift exit.

Lorenzo drove me into work. In the car, I asked him about why this person had been gleefully quizzing us so much. It turned out he'd told her about my job. I felt sick. He hadn't discussed this with me first or even given me a heads-up. It was a total betrayal and made me feel incredibly vulnerable to the vultures and bullies who felt they had the right to publicly shame and taunt me because they found out that I was a sex worker.

I had so far kept my circle of friends small. It was easier to know who to trust when I spent pretty much all my time with colleagues from work. So, to be in a different group of people and to be challenged about my movements in such a condescending way came as quite a shock. It made me realise that I really had to be very careful about who I chose to have in my inner circle. It's not like I hadn't been aware of the stigma around the job I did, but the loaded questions from this woman showed that judgement could come in many forms. She seemed to have seen it as something she could use against me, like a power play.

• • •

A couple of months after I began dating Lorenzo, I reluctantly took my trip up Australia's east coast. I had been so excited to plan the trip and it had been one of my reasons for taking the job, but now it didn't feel right to be leaving. I was starting to really find my feet with living in Sydney. I was enjoying work and earning good money for the first time in my life. And, on top of that, I was falling head over heels in love with Lorenzo.

Even so, my trip up the east coast was an incredible experience. I went sailing around the Whitsunday Islands, scuba diving on the Great Barrier Reef, did a bungee jump in Cairns, visited crocodile farms and tasted crocodile for the first time. I met a fantastic group of people from all corners of the globe. I went on a trip to Fraser Island, the famous sand island with its population of dingoes. I saw so many beautiful places and created memories to last a lifetime.

But I missed Lorenzo. I was about halfway through my trip when I received a message from him to say that he couldn't see me anymore. I was absolutely heartbroken. I couldn't understand why; things seemed to be going so well between us. He gave no explanation – it was all so sudden and out of the blue. For the rest of my trip, I had a cloud hanging over me. There were some fun times but I just could not shake off the hurt I was feeling.

While I was in Cairns, my final stop before flying back to Sydney, Katie messaged me and asked me if I would like to move in with her. I was so excited and happily said yes. I had been worrying about where I was going to live on my return. I had moved out of the hostel in Coogee Beach and really didn't want to go back to sharing a room with two other people.

I later returned to Sydney ready to move in with Katie but was still feeling heartbroken. Katie very kindly picked me up from the airport. While we were in the car, she began telling me about this guy she'd met at work and how dreamy he was and how well they connected. My heart began to sink – the man she was describing sounded just like Lorenzo. I asked her if he had any distinctive tattoos. Yes, she said, and began to describe the tattoo on Lorenzo's forearm. 'Yep, that's my ex,' I said, feeling totally defeated. Katie soon messaged him and confronted him. A true friend.

Lorenzo had never shown any signs of having an issue with my job. I had thought everything was going well with him. But we did end up chatting one day after the break-up and it turned out that yes, he did have an issue with it. He claimed that he would have 'gone mad' had he started really falling in love me while I was doing that job. But still, he dropped me suddenly and then started pursuing my friend Katie, who did the exact same job. So I didn't know what to believe. Either way, it was perhaps an early warning sign about the perils of dating clients. If so, it was one I completely failed to heed.

∙ ∙ ∙

Living with Katie and a couple of the other ladies from work felt like being part of a real sisterhood. Jo was a total beach babe, who loved to get stoned and hang out by the beach. Camila was a voluptuous Latina with baby-blue eyes that had an ability to hypnotise and lure in just about anybody who dared to look. And then of course there was my friend Katie, a New Yorker who just oozed vibrant energy.

I began to really soak up the Sydney social scene. Festivals, nightclubs, day clubs and boat parties became our thing, all we lived for. We just loved to party. Our main mission in life at that point was living for the weekend, chasing the next high. The more we went out, the more people we'd meet and we began to expand our social circle. The apartment, in Sydney's Inner West, was beautiful, with two huge balconies. We often hosted incredible afterparties, dancing on the balcony until sunrise, raising our hands in the air as the planes flew over en route to Kingsford Smith. We were having the time of our lives.

One evening, Katie walked in the door and announced that she had been invited to a friend's birthday party and she wanted me to come along. At the time, I was still pining over Lorenzo, but Katie convinced me that it would be good for me to get out. When we got there, the party was already in full swing. Katie had previously met Ethan on a night out in Kings Cross. His mates were a friendly bunch of guys, most of them tech geeks who knew each other from having studied IT together at university. We all connected.

Among the group was Ethan's good friend and business partner Jake. Jake was very down to earth and easy to talk to. And he shared the same desire to get high and party. He seemed very genuine. Jake had set up his business while studying at university. He came across as very driven but still had a calming energy about him. I felt safe around him.

One of my first impressions of Jake was that he would make a good husband, but that wasn't what I was looking for at the time. I liked that he didn't talk about other women as objects and there was something about him that felt very trusting. He wasn't like the rest of the guys in our social circle. He was less 'lads, lads, lads' and a lot more genuine and respectable.

We began dating. However, I did not tell Jake about my job. I made out that I had a lot of savings and my parents were also helping to fund my travelling. As we started to spend more time together and got to know each other better, I began to feel more and more guilty about Jake not knowing about my line of work. He made it quite easy for me to live a double life. He was one of those guys who just wasn't inquisitive. I could go out partying all night without him and he wouldn't call or message, not even once, to see how my night was going. He left me to do my own thing and didn't expect me to be constantly reachable. The nights I was working, I just said that I wasn't free that night and that would pretty much be it. He wouldn't ask any further questions. As far as he was aware, I had a lot of savings so didn't need to work.

Eventually, the guilt got the better of me and after a few months of seeing each other, I broke things off with him. It was a decision that I did not feel good about at all, but it did stop the guilt and the sheer exhaustion of having to live a double life. Initially I felt a sense of freedom, but then I began missing him.

I arranged to meet up with him. I felt that I wanted to explain to him in person the real reason why I broke things off. At least that way, he could make an informed decision about whether or not he wanted to be with me.

As we sat on Bondi Beach gazing out towards the glistening blue ocean, I began to explain: 'I wanted to meet up with you in person because I wanted to explain the real reason why I had to break things off with you.'

'OK,' he said curiously.

'I work in erotic massage.' I took a deep breath, hoping that he would not lash out.

CHAPTER FOUR
TWISTS AND TURNS

I continued to explain, 'The reason I broke up with you is because I just couldn't live with the guilt of not telling you but was worried about how you'd react.' I paused, waiting anxiously for his response.

The truth was I really didn't want to break up with Jake. I was falling in love with him. And that meant I didn't want to work at Tantra House anymore. The sheen of this fun and liberating job had been taken off by wanting to be with just one man. I am an 'all in' person, very loyal, and when I love, I love wholeheartedly. I had just learnt that my job was not going to be compatible with that.

But I was stuck. Firstly because I was so scared of his reaction, of him rejecting me, which was why it had initially felt less risky to call the whole thing off. But also, for the simple reason that the money at Tantra House was so good and so easily earned. I was ready to leave Tantra House on a high, to tone down the partying and spend more time with Jake. To be a couple. But at the same time, I had become used to a certain lifestyle and I still needed money to live, to pay my rent. My options for work were severely limited by the terms of my visa.

'Thank you for telling me,' Jake said calmly. It was immediately clear that he wasn't going to freak out or judge me. He was so understanding. My shoulders dropped and I felt my whole body relax. It was nice that he appreciated my honesty.

He had found the break-up hard, he said, and I guess from his point of view it must have been confusing: things were going so well with us, and then for no real reason, I'd broken things off. He had been very hurt.

I carefully explained that I wasn't ashamed of my job but I did feel that it wasn't something I could do any more if we were going to make a go of it. But that I needed to figure out what I was going to live on instead.

'I can help you get out of the industry,' he said.

'I would never expect that,' I replied. 'I just wanted to be honest with you. I felt that you deserved to hear the truth.'

'Thank you. But I'm sure I can help you,' he said.

'Thank you,' I said with all the gratitude in the world.

We hugged it out in the middle of the beach, holding each other tightly. I felt such a huge sense of relief. Like the biggest weight had just been lifted off my shoulders. The truth was out; I had told him that I was working in the sex industry and the world did not end. I took a risk being honest and this time, it paid off. I had enjoyed my time in the industry and was hugely grateful for it but was now ready to fall head over heels in love.

• • •

Jake and I continued living the high life; we still partied with the group, but also spent a lot of time together just the two of us. I started to organise group dinners so that we could do 'normal' things together, other than going out and getting trashed. He was supporting me financially while I was looking for another job. We were falling in love with each other. His calming energy soothed my wild ways and my bold and courageous energy boosted his confidence. This was the point at which Jake and I began building our lives together. I felt truly supported by him and his non-judgemental reaction about my line of work. It meant the world to me.

Camila had moved back to her home country and Katie was also planning to leave Sydney, so our sisterhood was beginning to disperse. The dynamics were changing. It was just Jo and I left.

During one of my dreaded trips to the immigration office to extend my visa, I was hit with a total shock when I discovered that I had stupidly overstayed. The immigration officer informed me that I needed to leave the country as soon as possible to avoid deportation. I would have to apply for a new visa while out of the country. Considering the situation, I was advised that it might take months, if it was even granted at all. My heart sank.

I had to accept the fact that I had to leave Australia and hold on to the hope that my visa would be extended and I could soon return to the happy life that I had created with Jake. So, I put on my 'big-girl pants', packed my bags, bit the bullet and returned home.

After living the high life in Sydney, I came crashing back down to earth with an almighty bang. I had to move back in with my parents at the farm and found myself back to clod picking in the pissing rain. How life can twist and turn! The situation put a huge strain on my relationship with Jake. I was well and truly stuck in no man's land, not knowing whether we had any sort of future. I felt incredibly lost. I was stranded in rural Bedfordshire while my heart and soul remained in Sydney.

...

It was early 2008, and I had been living back at home for almost six months. Jake had managed to come and visit over Christmas and during that time we both travelled to Germany to meet his parents at their holiday home. But still, it was a real struggle being apart and not knowing when I would return. Saying goodbye to him at the airport was excruciating. We had no choice but to hang on to the hope that we would be back together in Sydney soon.

That day couldn't come soon enough in my mind. I was not getting on with my parents at all. For work, I was doing jobs on the farm for my dad as well as working in a local village pub. But I was sad and preoccupied; I just did not want to be in Bedfordshire. My parents didn't really understand and the tension grew.

Eventually my mum and dad told me I had to move out. In a panic, I packed up my things, booked a taxi and headed straight to the train station. Luckily, a friend knew of a pub in north London looking for bar workers and offering accommodation so at least I was able to quickly put a plan in place.

My first experience of living in London at twenty-four years old was tough. I had visited a few times but never lived there and the only people I knew in the capital were my Aussie friends – Katie from New York was now there, thankfully, and another friend from Sydney, Isla. I moved in to the pub but the guy I was working for was a total dick, so I ended up moving to a youth hostel in west London. I was living on the breadline, making money from temping here and there. Asking my parents for financial help was a bigger no then ever considering the state of our relationship – we weren't even communicating.

My pride wouldn't allow me to ask Jake for financial help either. Our relationship was straining under the pressure of being so far apart for so long and not knowing when or even if we'd ever see each other again. So I also feared that asking him for money would only make things worse. I was working with an immigration lawyer who was trying to help me with my visa application so I could get back to Sydney, but because I'd overstayed my visa it was very difficult and there was no guarantee that I'd be able to return, ever. It was a waiting game that left me stuck in limbo. All I could do was be patient and stay positive.

It got to the stage where I didn't have enough money for tampons and had to resort to using toilet paper from the youth hostel. To be living in the capital with nowhere else to go made me feel very vulnerable. I was overwhelmed.

Naturally my mind turned to sex work. I began to search for erotic massage companies. There were no venues, not like in Sydney. I had no idea how these things worked in London. What I did find on my search was outcall and incall agencies, 'incalls' meaning the client comes to wherever the masseuse is, outcalls meaning that the masseuse visits the client. Considering I was sharing a room with five other ladies all sleeping in bunk beds, outcalls to the client in hotels was my best option. Somehow, I didn't think my roommates would have appreciated clients coming in and out of the room for a massage and a happy ending ...

If I was going to do this it meant lying to Jake. I just knew that I couldn't tell him. I didn't feel good about it and I knew that it would weigh on my mind, but I was in survival mode. Other options felt thin on the ground.

After applying to a few erotic massage agencies, I received a response from Erotica Massage. I arranged a meeting with a lady from the agency at a coffee shop close to Kensington High Street. She was tall and graceful and had an air of mystery about her. When I asked her where she was from, she replied, 'Up north' – my first real lesson in discretion (and one I probably could have done with heeding a little better). We sat opposite each other, with the din of London on the other side of the door, and she began to ask me questions about my previous experience. To outsiders, we probably looked like a pair of colleagues having a regular meeting in a coffee shop dressed in our corporate wear. But to each other we were testing the waters, trying to unpeel the layers, deciding if we wanted to collaborate in a world where the lines between business and pleasure are blurred.

After the interview, I headed back to the hostel to digest it all. I was unsure about how it had gone. My interviewer had given very little away and left me feeling doubtful that she wanted to take me on. However, a couple of days later, I received a text welcoming me to the team. A huge weight had been lifted. *An end to my money worries*, I thought. Overjoyed, I gladly accepted. My return to the world of erotic massage began.

• • •

Working for this agency was my first taste of working high-end in London. One afternoon, I received an outcall booking to the Dorchester. At twenty-four, I had no real clue about this hotel or how iconic it was. I got out of the cab and entered the most imposing, jaw-dropping hotel reception, complete with marble flooring, I had ever laid eyes on. It was so very *shiny*. Dressed in subtly sexy corporate wear, I teetered along in my high heels and tried my best not to fall over or create a scene. Avoiding eye contact with reception, I discreetly made my way to the lift.

When I arrived at the client's hotel room, I knocked loudly enough so he could hear me but not so loudly as to attract attention from neighbouring rooms. A middle-aged man who appeared to be of Middle Eastern descent opened the door, all smiles, warm and friendly. I knew instantly that we'd get along and so my body immediately relaxed. After brief introductions, I asked the client to sort the 'formalities' so we could then focus on relaxing and having some fun. Once I'd counted the cash and was happy that the amount was correct, I slipped it into my purse and asked the client where the bathroom was so I could change into my lingerie. The client showed me the bathroom and left me to it.

To this day, I don't think I've ever seen such an impressive bathroom: shiny marble flooring, his and hers sinks, the fluffiest of fluffy dressing gowns. Classic, stylish, oozing with elegance. The bedroom itself was huge, with the most comfortable king-sized bed taking centre stage. I slipped out of the bathroom, fully transformed in stockings, suspenders and stilettos, and headed over to the bed where the client was eagerly waiting for me. My massage skills had progressed slightly from the early days of Tantra House when I had no idea what I was doing, but I was still learning. This client liked to chat so I felt comfortable around him. As I slathered his body in oil, massaging his back and shoulders, we chatted about food, about London and the fine restaurants that it had to offer. I had learnt to really build up the massages, to tease the client to the point of them begging me to wank them off. This client was no exception. Being a tease became my signature style. Before I knew it, the client had blown his load and I was out the door heading down to reception to get a cab back to my six-bunk room at the youth hostel.

Most of my bookings were done in and around Kensington, Chelsea, Knightsbridge and Mayfair. Such beautiful parts of London, rich in history, with beautiful architecture. I felt such a sense of old romance in this part of town. Some of the homes and hotels I visited were out of this world and unlike anything I had ever experienced before (again, all marble, all shiny). It was a far cry from my early experiences at Tantra House and felt like a step up in the world. The clientele was different too – more professional, suited and booted, lots of business travellers, and not the mix I had been used to. Looking back, I did not appreciate how fortunate I was to be working in these areas because at the time, all my focus was on returning to the life that I had built in Sydney.

I was soon booked on my first duo outcall, which meant the client had requested two of us. She was stunning – a Latina with curves in all the right places; toned, beautiful with long, dark hair. I was totally mesmerised by how natural and in the moment my duo partner was. While the client was laid flat out on his back, she straddled over him, sitting on his stomach with her back to him (I was demoted to foot massager). As she slowly caressed his penis, she threw her head back and let out the most erotic and breathy 'aaaaa', with her back perfectly curved and her glossy locks shimmering under the light. I felt hypnotised by her beauty and sexuality and confidence in her own body. From this booking I learnt so much about taking your time, about being present and in control. She had the client right in the palm of her hand (come to think of it, she had us both in the palm of her hand!). I don't know if she really was, but it was so convincing that she was enjoying herself. She inspired me. The best way of learning as a sex worker was to observe others; what to do and what not to do.

I soon found it obvious when a colleague was being fake with a client and just wanted him to cum as quickly as possible so she could leave. The client would sense it and I would sense it. I made sure that I never made a client feel that way. I had of course picked up techniques from my work in Sydney – not necessarily deliberately, but if I saw one of the ladies do something that worked, I'd make a mental note and perhaps try it out myself. However, the experience with my first duo partner had a lasting effect on me and served as a 'how to' for future bookings.

• • •

The money I was earning meant my financial worries were no longer burning away at the back of my mind every waking moment, so in that respect, things were better. But my relationship with Jake was not. I couldn't bring myself to tell him what I was now doing for work. We were already arguing a lot, then we'd make up, argue, break up and then make up again. Our relationship was under a huge amount of pressure. I had my suspicions that he had been unfaithful. No proof, just a hunch. He was still out partying, doing drugs, living the high life, while I was living on the breadline in a hostel, having just been kicked out of my family home. I wanted to be back in Sydney, but still it rankled that he'd never even considered moving to the UK with me. It was all about Australia and his work, his friends, his family. I began to resent him for that.

But then a few months later, in the summer, Jake came to visit me in London. He proposed to me on the London Eye. Getting married was something that we had previously discussed when Jake suggested it during one of our phone calls. When he had first brought it up, I wasn't sure. I lost count of how many times I changed my mind. I was still only twenty-four and had never really dreamt of marriage. I was never one to make a half-arsed decision; if I said yes to something, it was because I meant it. I couldn't be fake. But even though I didn't feel ready to get married, I recognised that it was the only way for us to be together. I loved him and the distance was putting us under so much pressure. So when Jake went down on one knee while overlooking the London skyline, I happily accepted.

I finally returned to Australia in September 2008. I could not wait to pick up where I left off and continue to build the life that I loved with Jake. It had been a year of putting my life on hold in the UK, not knowing what lay down the road, so I was ready to put that all behind me and move on. Before leaving the UK, I ensured that I patched things up with my parents. I did not want to return to the other side of the world with such negativity hanging over us.

If I was expecting to go straight back into the crazy partying that I'd left a year ago, I soon discovered that a lot had changed. The group we once partied with were beginning to slow down as they got into life in the corporate world post-uni. The nights out weren't on the crazy scale that they had been before. But none of that really mattered – I was just ecstatic to be living back in Sydney and for Jake and I to be living together as a couple once again.

Jake and I got married on 23 April 2009 on a jetty in the Whitsunday Islands. Just the two of us. I had never dreamt of a big white wedding. I always knew that I would do things slightly differently if I ever decided to get married. We had a reception in Australia and also back home in the UK with my friends and family so that we could still all celebrate.

Shortly before getting married, I had begun my journey into corporate life. At that point, I felt ready to be working in a 'secure' job with regular 9-to-5 hours. I started off working in customer services for an ATM company. I was able to hold that job down for a couple of years before the boredom got the better of me. The monotonous routine felt like it was crushing my spirit. Towards the end, I struggled to even get myself out of the car when I pulled up by the office. I felt a heaviness all over me. I would sit and stare aimlessly into the distance trying to pluck up the energy to get myself out of the car and to my desk, but my body was telling me no.

From there, I went into market research, which worked well for a time, but in the end it just felt like the same day unfolding over and over. The same soul-crushing, robotic routine moulding me into a well-oiled machine. Corporate life soon began to feel like I was stuck in a fishbowl, continually swimming around and around. I felt like I had no real meaning or purpose. What difference was I making to people's lives? How was I helping people on a personal level? I was questioning everything and began to disconnect. I became deeply unhappy.

Things got even worse when I went from market research to finance. I was the only woman working in a sales team of middle- aged men. I definitely got a lot less respect here than in sex work. One particular man in my team was so inappropriate, not just with me but with other women in the wider office. 'That's it, get down on your hands and knees,' he said to one girl who was bent down by the photocopier. He told our colleague, 'Stick Elizabeth in a short skirt and send her off to the sales conference.' And there was another guy in our team who was also weird and pervy, and would sometimes greet me in the office with a kiss on the cheek. I felt so uncomfortable but was only young and did not know how to handle it.

It wasn't just in Australia that I had these experiences in offices. When I had been temping in London I was sitting at the reception desk of one company and a male colleague walked in one morning and said, 'Your tits look great in that top.' I was too shocked to say anything but I did inform the temp agency. They had already received complaints from others who were sent there before me, yet they carried on sending young women there anyway, making no effort to address the issue.

By contrast I had found sex work empowering because it was all on my terms; I was in control and, at work, far from being looked down on, I got respect. Working in an office, it was the men who called the shots, and that included perving on us. It was often a weird power play, I noticed. However uncomfortable we felt, there was almost nothing we could do about it.

When I did end up complaining about the inappropriate behaviour of a colleague, I was fired.

Luckily, I had started pursuing a passion of mine – acting. There was an acting school only a short walk from where Jake and I lived in a leafy neighbourhood of Sydney. I began with the drop-in classes and then started committing to the short courses. It was my absolute ray of light during my corporate-life hell.

• • •

After almost six years together, Jake and I had begun growing apart. Looking back, I can see that it was almost inevitable when we had got married so young, before we really knew ourselves. I was starting to feel invisible to him and that he was taking me for granted. The sexual chemistry had completely gone and it just felt like we were two friends living together. The relationship began to lack connection and intimacy. He would often stay at work late to do drugs with his friends while I had moved away from that lifestyle. I wanted more from life.

We had planned to move to the UK together. Sydney was a special place where I held lots of treasured memories, but at that point, it just did not feel like home anymore. Australia had become a very lonely and isolated place for me. I was feeling the distance.

I wanted to be closer to my friends and family. I had squeezed every last bit out of Sydney, and there was nothing left for me. I had been accepted into acting school in London to study for a master's. A huge dream of mine was becoming a reality. But knowing how unhappy I was in our relationship, I just could not go through with it. I couldn't uproot Jake from all his friends and family, feeling as I did. As unhappy as I was, aside from asking my mother if I was adopted, it was one of the most difficult conversations I have ever had.

'What do you think about having a trial separation?' I said to him one evening on the couch.

'I sensed something was wrong when we were in Fiji,' he said. He had thought something was wrong when we were on holiday? But this was months ago. 'Then why didn't you say anything?' I asked him, completely baffled by his statement.

'Because there is always the hope that things will get better,' he said.

My heart sank. But things did not get better – between us at least. So, with my new-found freedom, I flew back to London solo, ready to embark on a new chapter in my life.

CHAPTER FIVE
MONEY WORRIES

'And for God's sake, make sure your tuition fees are all paid, otherwise you won't be able to do your showcase!'

Those words stopped me in my tracks. It was term two of acting school and we were packing up after the end of another busy day. The tutor's words jolted me. I had been under the impression that we had until the end of the year to pay them. But the showcase was in September and it was now April. *Shit, shit, shit. Why didn't I pay the fees all in one lump sum at the beginning of the year when I had the finances?* Panic started to set in. The showcase was our chance to get the attention of London's top acting agents. It was a crucial part of the process and not doing it would have felt like the past year of gruelling work had all been for nothing. Well, that just wasn't going to happen.

I was fulfilling my dream of studying for a master's in acting at a highly accredited London acting school. I was twenty-nine and newly single, with the freedom to pursue my passion. I was exactly where I wanted to be at that point in my life. I had spent years fantasising about being on a London stage. Through sheer grit and determination, I was getting that master's no matter what. Nothing would stop me from achieving that dream. Not finances, not relationships.

I was also ecstatic to be living back on home soil after seven years in Australia. Towards the end of my time in Sydney, as I had started to face up to the reality that my marriage to Jake was not going to work, I had begun to long for the luscious green fields of the beautiful English countryside, blustery winter evenings sat in front of a roaring fire, British pub culture, greasy fish and chips, pie and mash, Sunday roasts with the family, British sarcasm. Basically, anything and everything that was quintessentially

British – you name it, I wanted it. I also felt the bright lights and buzz of London calling me. I could not wait to be living in a city that had theatres around every corner, being pushed and shoved in the morning rush, the Tube, black cabs.

My first week back home had been one of the happiest times of my life. I was so excited to be starting a new chapter in my life. As the plane bringing me home began its descent into Heathrow, I felt overwhelmed by the luscious green fields below. It looked like the most perfect patchwork. I could not help but shed tears of joy. I had never forgotten how beautiful England was. In fact, it was one of the things I had missed the most. I had so longed to reconnect with my roots. I really was a country girl at heart and had craved spending time in rural Bedfordshire. I could not wait to be on the farm again. Even though my family drove me a little crazy at the best of times, I came to the conclusion that I'd rather be living close to them driving me crazy than be without them.

As I came into the arrivals gate at Heathrow, there they both were, waiting patiently. 'Hi, Mum! Hi, Dad!' I said as I squeezed them both. I felt such relief to see them again. On the journey home, it was as if I was a newborn baby taking in my surroundings for the first time. I just could not stop gazing out of the window, taking in every little detail, from the British voices on the radio to the fields alongside the motorway. As we came into my home county, I was greeted with the most beautiful Bedfordshire sunrise I had ever seen.

I was so happy to be in London, learning about something I loved. But of course, studying for a master's was intense. The days were long and even when classes were over, we had studying to do at home in the evenings, which would often have me working until 1 a.m. This left barely any time for anything else – like earning money to pay the bills.

My parents did the best they could to help me out with a weekly allowance while I was at acting school. It wasn't enough but there was no way that I could ask them for money for my tuition fees as well. I hated any reliance on them at that point in my life and was constantly riddled with guilt. I'd taken my CV to all the local pubs and restaurants but heard nothing back. I'd also had a trial to be a 'shots girl' – someone who sells shots of alcohol to customers at their tables in bars – in Leicester Square, which went terribly wrong when the woman training me turned out to be a total bully.

I mulled over my options – or lack of – constantly. I was worried about how I would eat, about not having enough money to get to school, bills, rent and now the final instalment of my tuition fees, due nearly four months earlier than I had thought. When my tutor said those words in class an internal panic broke out. I had £5 to spend on food one week and had been living on a diet of nothing but rice and peas.

I carried those thoughts and worries around with me every day for weeks. The burden was beginning to feel heavier and heavier, the longer I put off dealing with it. I was racked with fear at the thought of not being able to pay my fees.

Don't get me wrong – I understand that this situation was all my own doing. I blame no one but myself. I didn't *have* to go to acting school in London; it wasn't a compulsory part of my education. But knowing what I do now, I can see that I didn't have the tools to manage my money. I was totally clueless. I hadn't been reckless with money – there was not much time for anything else other than studying, so having a wild social life was not even an option. But this isn't enough – you have to learn how to manage your finances too.

Some people are naturals, others are not and need time to learn.

While my parents must have spent a lot of money on things like our horses – my love of riding was certainly an expensive hobby – our lifestyle growing up was all about working hard on the farm and was in no way ostentatious. I was often told 'money doesn't grow on trees', which is helpful to no one! That was about the extent to which money was talked about at home.

When I was at university, my mum would open my mail from my bank, read my statements and give me a hard time for it. So, early on I was made to believe that I was 'bad' when it came to managing my money, which I now think only made the situation worse. I'm not blaming my parents; I'm sure my mum was just concerned and looking out for me. However, I cannot deny that these early experiences influenced my relationship with money.

Budgeting, mortgage rates, credit cards, APR, how best to save and ways to invest are just a few things that I (and many people!) have struggled to understand at various times. And I am definitely still learning. How much better life would be if we could be introduced to this stuff when we are young, before we start making mistakes! I absolutely think this is something that should be taught in schools – explaining everything so that it becomes crystal clear and sets up young people for the rest of their lives would be hugely beneficial. I give praise to Deborah Meaden for writing her book *Why Money Matters*, aimed at six- to nine-year-olds. We absolutely need to be seeing more books like this available in both primary and secondary schools.

What job would pay well enough and not interfere with my studies? I needed something more consistent that didn't require too much of my time so I could focus and fully immerse myself in my master's, but that still paid well enough so that I could get the remainder of my fees paid. Once again, I began to consider alternative ways of earning an income.

It's no surprise that so many students turn to the sex industry. Especially considering the rise in tuition fees and the burden of having to pay them off post-graduation. The sex industry offers a lot more pay for a lot less hours, more financial freedom and more time to study without having to go a day or two without food. Of course, the tabloids would depict this as young women being 'forced' into sex work, ignoring the fact that many in the industry have chosen this job because they want to do it, because the hours and the lifestyle works for them. No one should ever feel like they have no option but to do a job that they really don't want to do. If anyone does, then I think we should be questioning the cause of the economic disadvantages experienced by so many before blaming the sex industry for society's ills.

I have personally learnt a lot more about business and finances while working as a sex worker than I ever did at school, university or in the corporate world. Working in the industry taught me to manage my finances better, to start investing and growing my money, how to manage my accounts and pay my taxes, and to make my money work for me. Those lessons took many years to learn, but the sex industry is a hugely lucrative business, and the earning potential is there if used wisely.

ELIZABETH G.

• • •

Again, I tried searching for erotic massage venues but they were non-existent. I did find one in north London and went to see them, but as soon as I arrived I turned around and walked straight out the door. It was a shithole! There is no way I would have worked there. Then I tried Seeking Soulmates, which was a platform for 'sugar daddy' type arrangements.

A bit more of a grey area than sex work itself, which is much more clear cut and straight to the point. The general idea was that men and women alike could connect and set up mutually beneficial arrangements, such as a monthly allowance or 'pay per meets' in exchange for intimacy, a travel buddy, a dinner date. But the boundaries with this site were not clear and potential matches unreliable. I soon realised that this was not going to be the answer to my financial woes.

I started to think about escorting. I had only ever worked in erotic massage before. Yes, I'd had sex with some of the clients I'd met at Tantra House. But that was because I'd fancied them and I'd wanted to – not for money. Which is completely different. It felt like a big leap going from erotic massage to full service. But the more I thought about it, the more I started to realise it was a leap that I was willing to take. If it meant that I could focus on my studies, stop the sleepless nights, stop the worrying about money and get a weekly food shop in, then I would be happy.

As my money began to dwindle and the stress levels became unbearable, I began researching local escort agencies. I came across one agency, which I shall call Lust. Lust was based on the outskirts of London, not too far from where I was living at the time but far enough so that I wouldn't be working on home turf. I sent them an email detailing a bit about myself (age, hair colour, height, dress size, chest size, shoe size, etc.) and my experience working in erotic massage along with some photos and awaited their call. It was only a day or two later when I got my response: 'Can you come in for an interview?' Relief. I was in. All I needed was for the response not to be a no and I knew that I'd be able to handle the rest.

The office organised for a driver to come and pick me up and take me straight there for my interview and, potentially, my first day of work. It was happening. I did have my doubts about returning to the sex industry and felt nervous before what I hoped would be my first shift. I decided to start with a Sunday day shift as it fitted best around my studies. That morning, I packed up my bags complete with day dress, heels, condoms, lube, baby wipes, body spray and make-up. I told my housemates that I was off into town to visit friends. At that point, I was living with four other acting students who I hadn't really clicked with, so getting on with my own life separate from them was pretty easy. Still, I dressed in my 'civilian' clothes so as not to attract their curiosity.

I met the driver at my local tube station, his car model and registration already given to me by the office, and discreetly slipped in.

'Hi, how are you? Nice to meet you.' Obviously, I gave a fake name. The driver was friendly, and we clicked instantly. He had a calming energy so that helped me to relax and stay focused. After a forty-minute journey, we pulled up to the office. I took a deep breath.

I followed the driver up the outdoor staircase. He buzzed through to reception and the door opened. Security was tight. Lust was an outcall-based agency, so the sex workers visited the clients in their homes or hotels. There would always be a driver to take us to the client's location. The office was the base where both the drivers and sex workers could relax in between bookings, watch movies, eat, sleep and chat.

We walked through a lounge area complete with four or five large sofas and a widescreen TV. This was the ladies' lounge; the one for the drivers was separate. I walked in all smiles, saying hello. The ladies smiled back. My first impression was that it felt warm and friendly. Another sisterhood, I hoped. I followed the driver into the office, where there were two desks and a large map on the wall of London and the surrounds. I was introduced to the office manager, Kim, whom I felt instantly at ease with, which was a relief. I had already started to realise at this point that positive vibes and feeling at ease with colleagues is crucial when you work in the sex industry. I sat in front of her desk and we chatted. It was all very informal.

The interview was brief. Kim gave me an overview of the agency and how it all worked. There were two shifts: day shift and night shift. Day shift was 9 a.m. to 7 p.m. and night shift was 7 p.m. to 5 a.m. I was used to this from my days at Tantra House. There was no minimum number of days per week we were required to work. If we wanted to work one day a week that was fine and if we wanted to work five days a week, that was fine too. Most bookings took place in the London suburbs, or just outside the city limits in Buckinghamshire, Sussex, Kent, Surrey. I was told that I would be busy due to a lack of blonde English ladies.

I handed over my passport (presumably to check I could work in the country and potentially as some sort of safeguard against hiring trafficked women) and gave my vital stats so that a profile could be set up on the website. I'd decided to work under the name 'Emilia'. At some point I would need to get professional photos done, but initially, my selfies were sufficient. I chose not to have my face blurred out. I wanted to do whatever I could to ensure that I would be busy, and if that meant showing my face on the website then so be it.

I will always remember my first booking at Lust. It was around lunchtime that Sunday when the request came in. I had been booked with another female colleague. We were sent in separate cars (I would soon learn that, at the beginning of each shift, we'd be assigned our own designated driver for the day or evening to ensure efficiency) out to suburbia, arriving at a regular-looking, four-bed semi-detached. I felt insanely nervous. When we arrived, we were greeted by two good-looking men in their thirties, both high as kites, still up from partying the night before. I was not expecting that at all. I innocently assumed that a Sunday day shift would be pretty chilled. How wrong I was. As it was my first time, I was handed the money and I counted it in front of everyone. It wasn't until later, back at the office, that I realised I had counted the money wrong, and we were short. Fortunately, the owner of the agency was understanding and didn't let it affect my cut. I learnt from that mistake, and I never miscounted the money ever again.

All in all it was not the greatest first day. I could have done without the clients being so off their faces for a start. I could tell that my colleague wasn't particularly enamoured with them either, though she wasn't really the chatty, nurturing kind, so I was left to my own devices. But equally, I'd got it done and felt generally OK about it. I just had to trust that some bookings would be more relaxing in future! And many were. I was to meet some lovely clients while working for my first escort agency.

That evening, I couldn't tell anyone how my first day had been, as many people would after their first shift. No one in my life had any clue what I was doing. It's just one more facet of the stigma around sex work – other than our colleagues, we don't tend to have people we can talk to about our jobs. But at least I went home with a big wad of cash in my hand. I went straight to M&S to do a decent food shop. It was the most exciting supermarket shop I have ever done. Even today, when I've done my weekly food shop and unpacked it, I still find myself opening my fridge and standing in awe, feeling immense gratitude to have a fridge full of delicious, healthy food. It's something that I have never forgotten to be grateful for. To me, a kitchen full of food and a roof over my head is my life made because I know what it feels like to struggle and worry about getting money for the bare essentials. I do not take it for granted.

∙ ∙ ∙

At the beginning of each shift at Lust, the driver would pick me up from my requested location – I generally stuck to my strategy of choosing the nearest tube station as I didn't want my housemates spotting me getting into a car a couple of times a week right outside our house. I started working the 'graveyard' shift two nights a week. I'd leave my house 'plain clothed', telling my housemates that I was off out for the night to stay with friends in central London. And then off into the night I went to meet my driver, who would either take me to the office or straight to a booking. Going straight to a booking was always preferable as it meant I avoided getting too comfortable and sluggish in the office, ordering takeaway and falling asleep watching a movie.

Sitting in the lounge, I would wait until my name was called out over the speaker: 'Emilia, you have a booking.' Once called, I'd walk into the office and be handed a piece of paper with the client's name, number and location. I would then call the client. In the early days, I did not use a work phone so would call from my mobile and withhold my number. I would usually open the conversation: 'Hi, this is Emilia from the agency, are you looking for some company?' Once the client happily responded 'yes', I would continue. 'So it's a full sex service with a condom, no anal.' I would pause and wait for their response. If they were happy with that then I would continue with a description: 'I'm five feet five inches, dress size ten, natural 36DD bust, blonde hair, blue/green eyes.' And if the client sounded happy with my description, I would then confirm the price and ask for his full address and postcode. The piece of paper would be handed back to the office and a driver would be assigned. An ETA would be given, which always seemed to be around thirty minutes, given the easy access to the M25. If I wasn't dressed already, I would quickly nip into the toilets and transform from my casuals into dress and heels, and we'd be on our merry way.

Most of the drivers were great and I had fun chatting away and getting to know them. We'd share stories, have a laugh, turn up the tunes, head to McDonald's if we got the munchies. I loved being out and about on the open road. A good driver meant that the day or night would be a breeze. A minority of the drivers were not fit to do the job – it didn't happen to me but I did hear rumours that one had tried it on with some of the ladies. Others just did not seem bothered about our safety. Some were more interested in going to as many bookings as possible, regardless of our welfare. I didn't let this influence me. If I didn't want to go to a booking, I wouldn't go. Simple. If something didn't feel right or the client sounded too drunk or out of it, or just didn't vibe with me, it was a plain and simple no.

It didn't take long for me to make friends and build up my regulars at Lust. I got on well with the other ladies. As with Tantra House, they were from all walks of life, all ages, races, social classes. Single mothers, students, hedonists.

Jenny was a 'veteran' with many years of experience under her belt. She provided guidance for many of us who were new to the job. She was vibrant and energetic, smoked like a chimney and was always up for a party. She always had a funny story to tell. I will never forget how she told me about being on the Tube and her dildo falling out of her handbag and rolling all the way down the length of the carriage, to disapproving looks from the other passengers. Jenny was a true character.

'Party bookings' in escorting is essentially code for doing drugs, usually cocaine, with the client. Those ladies who were open to this would often have 'party booking' or simply the letters 'PT' on their profiles (other acronyms you might find on sex workers' profiles include 'DT', meaning deep throat, and 'DFK', meaning 'deep French kissing'. Further code names are 'PSE', meaning 'pornstar experience', which involves something of a mechanical, performance-style booking, and 'GFE', meaning 'girlfriend experience', which entails something more natural and relaxed). At that time, party bookings with fellow sex workers were always the preference. For one thing, clients were highly likely to extend the time allocated for the booking, which often meant staying in the same location all through the night with a client I'd built a rapport with, rather than being driven here, there and everywhere or waiting around back at the office. And of course they meant more money. And at the forefront of my mind was getting my tuition fees paid so that I could do my showcase. I knew what I had to do. I got my head down (quite literally) and worked my cotton socks off.

One of the most lucrative nights I had working at Lust was a party booking in suburban Berkshire. The booking started early, at 8 p.m., and went on all through the night and into the following day. My colleague and I left the client's house around midday, bleary-eyed and ready for bed. This particular booking remains clear in my mind because it was my first lesson in giving a client a prostate massage. The client had clearly done this many times before as he had a wooden rolling pin the length of my arm at the ready. As the drinks and cocaine flowed, music blaring, he urged me to insert the rolling pin. He positioned himself, backing up towards me on the bed on all fours. I knelt behind him. With the aid of lots and lots of lubrication, I slowly began inserting the rolling pin. Inch by inch, I watched in total amazement as the client urged me to continue: 'More, more, keep going,' he said. So, with his guidance, I continued inserting the rolling pin, higher and higher, until it almost disappeared. Even to this day, I've never witnessed anything quite like it. I still can't believe it was not painful for him. I remember him saying that he could almost feel the rolling pin just below his ribs. The thought of having an object like that so far inside makes me want to pass out. But that was his thing, and so as long as he was enjoying it, that's what mattered.

Time went by so quickly on cocaine. Night would easily morph into day and then back into night again. As morning appeared, the client's ex-wife decided to make a visit. He had already warned us that this might happen and assured us that they get on well enough and she would not be fazed to discover he had booked a couple of sex workers. But as soon as we heard her voice shouting up from downstairs, we instinctively grabbed our belongings and went straight into the bathroom, locking the door and leaving the client to chat with his ex. My colleague was freaking out but I was calm. I could tell by their conversation that they were friends, that she was understanding. 'Oh, have you got company?' I heard her whispering to him as I leant against the bathroom door, listening intently. Once she realised the situation, she swiftly exited – 'Have fun!'

By the time the booking finished, after about fifteen hours, I was well and truly ready for bed. The driver had been nearby in his car all night waiting for me, as they always did. I notified the office that the booking was about to finish and tried my best to discreetly slip out of the client's house and into the car, avoiding eye contact with any potential lurking neighbours. A quick change into my day clothes in the car and it was straight home from there. I did a quick count up, handing the driver his cut and also the cut for the office. In this particular instance, I got the driver to drop me off just a couple of streets away from my home. Once home, I slipped upstairs, jumped in the shower and went straight to bed.

During another day shift, I received a booking to visit a regular client of the agency, though he was not someone I had been to before. The driver and I pulled up to a very quaint-looking four-bedroom home in a pretty part of suburban London. I was greeted at the door by a man dressed in women's clothing. As I entered his home, I scanned the kitchen to see an array of empty beer bottles, plates of cocaine, rolled-up notes and a smoky haze. It was a Sunday morning and clearly he had not slept all night. In spite of this, I felt at home as he was very welcoming. We began to chat and immediately got on well. I was very curious and intrigued to hear his story. As we started to feel more at ease with each other, he began to tell me how he had opened up to one of his close friends about his desire to dress in women's clothing. The 'friend' did not take the news well and advised that he should go and talk to someone about it. He had been disowned by a number of his so-called 'friends' and as a result was alone and isolated just for doing what felt natural to him. He sought comfort in sex workers. It felt good to know that my presence in his life helped him. I did my best to help him embrace who he was and not to allow other people's judgement to affect him. They were never his friends in the first place, I told him.

Some evenings felt like a total breeze. I was soon beginning to build up my regulars. One of my favourites, whom I shall call William, was one of the kindest souls I have ever met. A true gentleman. Every booking, he would have a steaming-hot bubble bath ready and waiting for me. While I relaxed and soaked in the bath, he'd be downstairs in the kitchen cooking me a delicious meal. We'd sit and chat and connect over dinner followed by music and dancing in the living room and then a quickie in the bedroom. Nights like that I felt blessed. William lived alone and was just grateful for a woman's company and it really showed. As a result, I was always willing to go that extra mile for him.

Other shifts came with their challenges. It was early days and I was still learning. I was on a day shift when I was sent to a booking with the colleague with whom I'd done my very first shift. We pulled up to a modern-looking block of flats on the outskirts of London. As we entered the apartment, we were greeted by three men. To this day, I have never seen a group of men so wired; it was as if they had not slept for four days straight. They were so off their heads that their eyes were almost bulging out of their sockets like something out of a cartoon. Naturally, I was cautious, though I had the reassurance of my colleague, who, while not a natural nurturer, was incredibly streetwise.

My colleague ventured into the bedroom with her client, I remained in the lounge with mine while the third man hovered in the middle bedroom. There was no chitchat or getting to know each other with this booking. It was straight down to business. As I proceeded down on my knees, my head between the client's legs, out of the corner of my eye, I noticed two large machete knives.

Holy shit. Seeing those machetes triggered a surreal feeling. My mind and my body went into high alert on the inside but on the outside I remained totally calm. Cool as a cucumber. As though I understood that continuing to suck his cock was the best thing to do under the circumstances and the most likely thing to keep him stable. My current therapist has since explained my reaction as 'fawning' – I intuitively focus on befriending anyone who could be a threat, almost flattering them in order to keep the situation under control. My intuition is telling me not to panic or create tensions. Stay calm; don't let them detect my fear.

The client got up to get a drink and I felt that was my opportunity to go into the bedroom and casually and calmly tell my colleague that there were two whopping great machetes in the living room.

'He's got a fuckin' knife!?!' she exclaimed. She immediately went marching over to my client in the lounge.

I wondered what she was going to do but she submissively lay on her front, swaying her legs side to side with her head tilted and resting on her hand, looking up to him oh-so-sweetly. 'Why do you have a knife?' she said, as though she was a curious child.

'For protection,' he said unapologetically, eyes still everywhere as though he was King Kong surveying his estate. Protecting his land.

Somehow, we were able to finish the booking and made a very swift but calm exit, still being careful not to create any kind of hysteria or panic, or rock the boat in anyway whatsoever. Once out of the door, the pair of us must have looked like we had seen a ghost. Usually chatty and upbeat, we didn't say a word to each other as we left the building feeling like we'd just been given a second chance at life.

We took separate cars back to the office (as always, we were each assigned our own driver). Usually, I'd be chatting away to the driver or singing along to the music cranked up all the way back to the office. But this journey was different; I didn't say a word the whole way back. I was in total shock and disbelief as to the situation I had just willingly put myself in.

Luckily, this was a one-time occurrence and I have not had an experience like that since. I look back and am amazed at how calm I was. We all have our own coping and self-protection mechanisms. Staying calm, using my charm and playing the 'dumb blonde' around a potential danger is mine.

• • •

While nothing this frightening ever happened again, there were plenty more light-hearted escapades during my time at Lust. It was around this time that I was beginning to get quite familiar with the inside of a Premier Inn. During one of my night shifts, I was just heading out through reception, having just had a steamy session with a smoking-hot Essex boy, when reception texted me: 'Can you go back in? Another booking, room seventy-two.'

Shit, I thought. *Please don't be right next door to my previous client. Maybe the clients know each other? Maybe this is a set-up?* So many thoughts went through my head. The next booking wasn't next door, fortunately, but it was only a few doors down from the previous one. It turned out that the clients didn't know each other; it was just a massive coincidence. When I finished the second booking, I snuck out as quickly as I could and casually slipped into the car with the driver. Who had, by now, spent some considerable time parked outside the Premier Inn.

The shifts were long and could be exhausting. One day I was sent to a job somewhere on the south coast (we really did some mileage with this job!) in an immaculate four-bedroom home. I felt at ease; the client was very welcoming. We proceeded upstairs and got straight down to business. I could sense his balls were about to explode as soon as I walked through the door. In classic missionary (underrated in my opinion and by far the most popular!), he blew his load and, within an instant, passed out and went into a very deep sleep. It totally baffled me. I've never seen someone fall asleep so quickly.

I was exhausted. I had been working and studying non-stop. My batteries were running very low. The thought of having to strike up conversation or go for round two that day did not appeal to me (for one-hour bookings, I'd say around 50 per cent of clients would go for round two). So, always one to seize an opportunity, with thirty minutes still left to go, I did not move one inch for fear of waking the client up. I lay there still, not making a sound while the client – still on top of me, still inside me – snored his little head off. I became a human plank of wood.

I could just about see the clock on the wall over his shoulder. When the thirty minutes was up, I began nudging the client in a bid to wake him up. It did not work, so one big push and he finally awoke, dazed and confused. 'OK! Time for me to go!' I said. 'I'm just going to use your bathroom to freshen up.' And off I went.

• • •

I was starting to earn good money. Just one month in and my savings were gaining momentum, allowing me to start paying off my remaining tuition fees. I was out of the red. To me, it was a great balance; I'd work a couple of shifts a week and earn plenty to fund food, rent, bills and tuition fees. And best of all, the sex work was not interfering with my studies. If anything, it was enhancing them – I still firmly believe that roleplay, reading clients' body language, listening, intuition and adopting the character of 'Emilia' was hugely beneficial to my master's in acting.

During one of our group discussions in class, one of my classmates made a remark that made my ears prick up like a startled deer – 'Well, you wouldn't give Louie a blow job for £50,' she said, gesturing to our classmate. The tutor interrupted: 'Woah! That's a massive assumption. What about the single mother who has mouths to feed?' The tutor's response forced my classmate to stop and really think about what she had just said. To this day, I am hugely grateful to my tutor for challenging my classmate's judgement. In another life, I would have stepped in and said, 'Actually …' and gone on to explain that I was doing essentially that to fund my tuition fees. But I felt too much shame back then. It didn't feel like something I could speak about openly, and in light of remarks like my classmate's, it was no surprise why.

A rare night out had been organised with the whole class (it was a large group of around forty, divided into groups of three). We had been working so hard and getting our arses kicked left, right and centre by tutors pushing us to become the best actors that we could be. So, a night out on the town together was a welcome relief. As we staggered from one bar to another through the bright lights of central London, I linked arms with my good friend Freddie. Out of everyone in the group, I connected with

Freddie the most. We had clicked instantly and seemed to have a good understanding of each other. I don't know if it was the booze or feeling at ease with him or both, but as we walked arm in arm among the group, I proceeded to tell him about my profession as a sex worker. He was not fazed at all. I felt such relief; he was so understanding. Knowing that I had Freddie's support about a world judged by so many meant everything.

Looking back over the years, I have found it hard to know who to trust enough to tell about my profession as a sex worker. Not everyone has been as understanding as Freddie. Friendships have come and gone, though the solid ones have remained. Reactions have been mixed. Some people have been supportive, some haven't. Some have become curious and asked if the agency is looking for more ladies. Others have lashed out and used it against me. A real mixed bag.

A common experience I have had is that someone seems fine with it at first but then, over time, their underlying issues with it become apparent. The cracks start to show. There has been a lot of prejudice or unconscious bias at the very least. This can be very hurtful when it's coming from my 'friends'. A lot of the time, I don't think they could even see themselves just how judgemental they were being.

'You really shouldn't,' was one very angry response.

'Just don't tell them details of your job,' said another, while I was discussing the possibility of telling friends within our group – advising secrecy and, therefore, implying that I should feel shame.

'Don't worry, I've not told anyone your secret!' That seemed to be almost taunting me, as if they had something over me, some sort of power.

Others have used it as a way to openly put me down and discredit me – 'fucking whore'. So naturally over the years, I have learnt to keep it to myself. You really need to prove yourself as a person before you reveal to people that you are a sex worker, I have discovered. This needs to change. Even today, it's a huge risk for anyone working in the adult industry to tell others about their profession.

One recurring theme I started to notice as I got into my thirties and I knew more people with children was an underlying resentment from unhappy women and mothers who tried to indirectly punish me for the decisions that they'd made. They have come across as bitter and jealous of the freedom and financial independence I have created without even thinking about all the sacrifices I have made along the way. I've never punished them for having the security of a family, so why try to punish me for a decision that they made? Is this something that all single, financially independent women feel to a degree? And is this heightened when they know I am a sex worker, seemingly an easy category to place in a box and judge harshly? Perhaps through me they see the life they could have had – the independence, the freedom to grow into their true selves. I guess in some ways they do resent me for that.

'You don't have any responsibilities!' is one thing I have been told. Sure, because sex workers just lounge around in their lingerie all day playing with their hair and filing their nails? If only!

So I have learnt to keep my circle of friends small. I feel like a certain level of isolation is inevitable if you work in the adult industry in the social climate we have today. I had to protect myself. I've learnt to only allow room for kind, trustworthy and compassionate people in my life. Compassion is everything.

I am so grateful for the friends who have accepted my profession and in turn accepted me as I am, without allowing it to become an issue and get in the way of our beautiful friendship. These friends are my little treasures.

• • •

My confidence had grown a lot since that nervous first shift at Lust, but in any job where you are dealing with people and human behaviour on a day-to-day basis, strange things can happen.

I remember in particular one daytime booking. I was dressed as discreetly as I possibly could be while at work – heels and a knee-length dress. The location was your average middle-class housing estate. The driver dropped me off and I headed towards the front door, trying not to attract attention, while the driver waited close by for the all-clear. The door began to open but there didn't seem to be anyone there. I looked down in horror to see that a small child had opened the door. I was mortified and started legging it in the other direction. But before I knew it, a woman came out of the house and was chasing after me. I was in a total panic and just wanted to get in the car and as far away as possible. But as I turned, I saw that the woman following me was smiling. She appeared understanding, as if this situation had happened many times before.

It turned out that this exact situation *had* happened many times before, with the two addresses often getting mixed up. She cheerfully pointed me in the right direction. When I did arrive at the correct address, I was greeted by a lovely man who was wheelchair bound. I explained to him what had happened and we both laughed it off. I am grateful to the lady who chased after me knowing full well what was going on, without judgement. Thank you, kind lady.

I tried to be more discreet for daytime bookings because of situations such as the above. We were expected to wear a dress and heels to every booking but some of us ignored that 'rule' and dressed in a way that made us feel more comfortable. Discretion was always the key for me. I would dress in a way that attracted the least amount of attention but still made enough effort so that the client would be happy.

My preferred driver was always Phil, a true Londoner through and through. I had a soft spot for him. We shared the same sense of humour and always had a lot of fun together out on the road. I knew I could trust him in any situation – such as one that involved a client running out of the door half naked in the middle of the day, leaning down towards the passenger side, begging me to stay. Phil responded admirably quickly when I said, 'Go, Phil, go, drive, drive! Get me out of here! That's why I had to leave.' Flooring it as fast as he could away from the client, who turned out to be more of a liability than I could deal with, we laughed our heads off. 'Bloody 'ell!' he said.

It must have given the neighbours quite a show. The client had tried everything to get me to stay, including offering me extra cash, but after being with him all through the night, I was weary and ready for bed. Even back then in the early days, I knew my limits. I wasn't totally driven by money – that's what kept me safe, physically and mentally. I wasn't willing to do anything with anyone. Enjoyment of the job was just as important as the pound notes.

ELIZABETH G.

A client who would soon become a trusted regular was 'Mr Sassy'. This particular client was turned on by humiliation and loved having his cock secured in a lock and being called every degrading name imaginable while wearing ladies' underwear. In the early days, humiliating clients was something that took me some time to get used to as it is not in my nature to be that way. But the more he encouraged me, the more my confidence grew. I enjoyed visiting Mr Sassy. He lived in a plush part of Surrey and we seemed to get along well. The chemistry just worked. He would often book for multiple hours and, more often than not, all the attention was on him. It wasn't uncommon to visit mega mansions in some of the plushest parts of suburban London. It was nice to be surrounded by the finer things, but it didn't always equal the best bookings. It always came down to chemistry.

Another booking that still stands out in my mind nearly ten years later was in a pretty part of Kent, a rural village with a stone bridge running over a quaint little stream. I arrived through an archway to the car park of a block of modern-looking flats. As I got out of the car, I was greeted by the client's grandmother who (quite surprising to me) had arranged the booking. She seemed like a lovely, kind, sweet-natured lady – straight away I felt her warmth and empathy. She smiled sweetly as she passed me the money. 'Have fun!' she said and walked in the other direction, leaving me to it.

I headed to the ground-floor apartment, where the door was open. As I entered, I walked towards the bedroom where I saw the client lying on the bed. A very handsome man in his thirties. He was disabled. His grandmother had explained the situation over the phone, so I half knew what to expect. He had previously been in a motorbike accident, which had left him unable to walk, but he still had some use of his hands and an ability to speak in slow speech. I always remember this client – so incredibly handsome, but more than that it was his energy. It makes me think of that famous quote from Maya Angelou: 'People will forget what you said, people will forget what you did, but people will never forget how you made them feel.' That could not have been truer of this booking. As I began to remove my bra, his eyes lit up with total glee, almost popping out of his head. To this day, I have never seen someone so excited to see my breasts. I wish I had stayed in contact with him. I have never met a more kind, genuine, lovable, gracious client. And what an understanding grandmother he had!

It was bookings like these that made the job all worth it. Clients like this one are reminders of why I do the job. It really isn't as many assume it is. Most days I feel more like a therapist than anything else. It really is helping people. It's the 'feel good' service. It's listening to people, being present with people, leaving all my crap behind to focus on someone else. It's about having energy and being positive. It's about putting on a smile and showing the best parts of me. That is what the client pays for. The most professional of sex workers understand this.

Another booking that stands out was with a man who only a few weeks earlier had lost his brother to suicide. He just wanted a massage, nothing else. Just a regular massage. I could feel in his energy the need to connect and be nurtured. He was absolutely in good hands. As a natural nurturer and empath, I have a way of helping clients to heal. I'm totally dedicated to making clients feel their best after their booking, and this particular client was no exception.

I have seen so many clients over the years who are mentally going through a very tough time. What better way to overcome life's challenges than to spend time with another human, chatting and having sex, feeling skin on skin, connection and energy? That's what sex work is really about. It's about a connection between two consenting adults. It's about expressing care and healing. If it was just about sex then the client would be watching porn and masturbating. It's more than that. Connection is what clients are really wanting, whether they know it or not.

Looking back, my experiences at Lust were a crucial part of developing my skills as a sex worker. The jobs and clients were very varied. Some were fabulous, some mediocre. It taught me stamina, resilience and the art of playing the character of Emilia.

• • •

I had been working at Lust for about four months when I received a certain booking request. 'Emilia!' My name was called on the loudspeaker. I walked into the office and Kim handed me the details. 'Shaun in Ilford.' I picked up my phone and sat in the private room to make the call.

'Hi, Shaun, it's Emilia from the agency. How are you?'

'Very well, thanks, darlin', how are you?'

'I'm really good, thank you. Are you looking for some company?'

'Yes, darlin', I am.'

'Would you like a description?'

'OK ...'

'I'm five feet five inches, long blonde hair, naturally busty 36DD, dress size ten.'

'Nice.'

'Do you have any questions about the service?'

'Nope, I just *love* licking pussy,' he responded with great enthusiasm. I felt relief that for one booking, I could relax and be pleasured. It was music to my ears.

'OK, that's fine. I don't mind that,' I said, half giggling. 'So it's a full sex service with a condom, no anal.'

'OK.'

'Would you like to book?'

'Yeah, babe, how long will it take you to get here?'

'I'll be there in about thirty minutes. Can I just get your address?'

The booking was made. I grabbed my bags and jumped in the car with Peter, another of my favourite drivers. He was great; laidback and not at all pervy, which was always a bonus. We would often have stimulating and intellectual conversations. We had recently talked about the negative side to taking drugs. A couple of weeks prior, I had been in hospital with angina after doing far too much cocaine over my birthday and at work. A scary experience. It was enough to put me off drugs, for now. Peter told me that he had lost a few friends to drugs. One had a heart attack and the other a brain haemorrhage, both due to taking cocaine. They were only in their forties. It scared me to death and made me think twice about doing drugs in the future.

As we drove into Ilford and approached the address of the booking, we passed some dodgy-looking flats. *Oh God*, I thought to myself, *not a dodgy booking in a rundown flat. I have a bad feeling about this one; it's going to be awful.* As we approached the building, I was pleasantly surprised.

It was a converted warehouse-style block of apartments. Pristine condition with high floor-to-ceiling windows. We pulled in to the private car park and I breathed a sigh of relief. My sense of foreboding had, unusually, been wrong. I was looking forward to going in and meeting Shaun.

Peter pulled up right outside the front doors.

'See you soon, Peter,' I said.

'Have fun!' he replied.

I made my way up to Shaun's apartment, knocked on the door and waited.

'All right, darlin!' He was tall with broad shoulders and strong arms. I was greeted with the cheekiest grin and a vibrant energy. He seemed genuinely happy that I was there.

'Hi, I'm Emilia,' I said as he closed the door behind me. Perhaps if I'd known in that very moment what his true intentions were, I may never have walked through that door.

CHAPTER SIX
CRAZY LOVE

* Trigger warning: domestic violence *

Shaun and I had clicked instantly and he'd become a trusted regular. This led to us exchanging numbers and seeing each other outside of the agency, breaking a general rule with Lust that we were not to meet up with clients privately. In terms of looks, he wasn't my usual type, but when the chemistry felt that good, I just couldn't help wanting to be in contact with him. We'd talk, drink, dance, snort cocaine (all my resolutions after my experience of having to go to hospital had been forgotten) and have great sex; it all felt so easy.

It was August 2013 and the summer vibe in London was in full swing. I felt like I'd hit a really exciting time in my life. My tuition fees were paid and my focus was all on my showcase in September, which would hopefully lead to getting signed with an agent and full-time acting work. I was almost there. I had worked so incredibly hard at my master's; now, after years of dreaming of working as a professional actor in London, my time was here. I felt ready.

My good friend Katie from New York, who had been living in London, was preparing to move back home to the States. I was sad to see her go but I had decided to take over her tenancy in her one-bed flat in Hampstead, north London. I felt very drawn to this vibrant and affluent part of London. Charming period properties lined the streets with terracotta pathways leading to large front doors. In springtime the many cherry trees came into full bloom with the most beautiful pink blossom. It was an area never short of somewhere to eat, drink or get a beauty treatment.

After a year of living in a student house, I was more than happy to be moving out and into a place of my own. So much so that I left a month before the tenancy had finished.

I loved finally having my own space. The bedroom was beautiful, with an old fireplace and large window looking down on the garden where the squirrels would play. For the first time in my life, I had my own place and full independence. I was incredibly happy and excited for the next chapter in my life. I no longer had to sneak around when going to and from work. I was able to come and go as I pleased without having to make up some crap and worry about being interrogated by my housemates. I was looking forward to enjoying the summer, putting more shifts in with work and getting myself ahead.

There had been just one red flag early on with Shaun, but I brushed it away. After one of my early bookings with him, he'd texted me to tell me that I had left a five-pound note at his. 'It's not mine so you keep it,' I replied. I knew that I hadn't left any money behind; I was always very careful wherever I was not to leave anything, especially money. I always had a sixth sense for things like that even when I had been drinking.

'No, it's definitely yours, babe, I will give it to you when I see you next.'

It was seemingly a tiny thing, yet my instincts were telling me that it was a bit strange for him to be so persistent about this bloody five-pound note. Looking back, I am sure that was his way of ensuring that he would see me again. His way of implementing some control.

We'd been spending more and more time together. Then, one early Sunday morning, I checked my phone and saw I had nine missed calls from Shaun. Luckily, I had put my phone on silent. He called again and I picked up. 'Hi, darlin', you all right? I'm coming to see ya!'

I was exhausted, I had been working all through the night, but he was so persistent and his energy so infectious that eventually I gave in. He ended up staying with me for five days straight. We spent most of that time in bed, having sex, ordering takeaway, watching movies or going out for dinner in Hampstead. It was heaven. One day, with my head resting on his chest and his big strong arms wrapped around me, a great big grin on his face and sweat glistening from his forehead, he said to me, 'I'm so happy.' I will never forget that moment. I really felt the meaning of those words.

'Me too,' I replied. I could not have meant it more. It was such a happy and perfect time in our lives. We were falling head over heels in love with each other. We were ecstatic to have found each other and to be living in this fantasy-like dream world. In that moment, nothing else seemed to matter.

'Have I told you how beautiful you are today?' he'd say.

'Nope,' I'd say, smiling like the Cheshire Cat.

'Well, you are very beautiful! Have I told you how much I love you today?'

'Nope,' I'd say again.

'Well, I love you very much,' he'd say with his eyes locked on mine.

My heart beamed with love. I had never felt so incredibly special and loved in all my life. All the insecurities I had from never feeling good enough, never feeling loved enough, never feeling special enough were gone, completely eradicated from my life. He made me feel like no man had ever made me feel before. I didn't think love like this existed. I never for one minute questioned it. He loved me and I loved him and that was all that mattered. *So long as we are together, we will always be happy*, I thought. It was intense and passionate and made me feel more alive than I had ever felt. He promised me safety and security like no one ever had. And above all, he believed in my acting ability, and that meant the world to me.

He would buy me flowers and drive me everywhere, telling me that my days of getting the train were over. He took me out for dinner, promised holidays, promised the world and put me high up on a pedestal. 'Let me look after you,' he'd insist. 'You've got to let me in your life, let me take care of you. We are going to have a great life together!' he'd say so convincingly. I was still working at Lust when I first started dating Shaun. It must have been hard for him but he didn't use it against me at the time. I felt so lucky that he was so understanding. Little did I know that one day that would all change.

One evening, Shaun organised to pick me up from the theatre. I went to see *The Herd* with a friend from acting school. Obviously, I had my phone on silent during the play. When the play finished, I checked my phone to see that I had nineteen missed calls from Shaun. It didn't freak me out. All I thought was, *Wow, this guy is really keen, he must really like me.* Fast forward to today and knowing what I know now – a bombardment of phone calls is a massive red flag. If you are in this situation, I advise you to run as fast as you can in the opposite direction and never look back. This never occurred to me. This man was treating me like a queen.

Another evening, Shaun and I had been to see one of my fellow actors in a play. Shaun loved it. Shortly after though, we got into an argument. I saw him flirting with one of the actresses at the bar and got upset. So we soon left. 'I knew this would happen,' he said, starting to panic that I would break up with him. He started banging his head against a doorway aggressively. It scared me; I had never seen him like this before. I was confused. I insisted that we walked back to mine. Once home, we sat and talked.

We were both anxious. I'd just had two weeks off work and was set to go back the following evening. I didn't want to. I was dreading it. The past two weeks with Shaun had been heaven and the thought of having to touch and be intimate with another man made me feel physically sick.

'You've got to let me help you out,' Shaun said, referring to his offer of financially supporting me. 'I don't want you to go back to work.'

'I don't want to go back to work either,' I said.

'Then let me help. I love you and want to be with you. I want to support you and help you out with your acting,' he said.

It felt so wrong to be going back to work but so right to be with Shaun. So, eventually, after much persistence on his part, I accepted his offer.

The following day while we were out on the Heath, I made the call to work. 'I won't be able to work for you anymore. Thanks for everything.'

'OK, Emilia, anytime you want to come back, you are always welcome.'

And that was it. We celebrated with dinner and drinks. I was so happy and excited about our future together. It just felt right.

ELIZABETH G.

While out driving through London one morning, with Stevie Wonder blaring through the speakers, windows wide open and beeping his horn, Shaun started shouting to passers-by: 'This is my girlfriend, she's the bollocks! I love her!' Over and over. People just smiled and laughed. I had the biggest grin on my face. At that point, I just could not imagine life without the man who was prepared to shout out about his love for me through the streets of London. It felt stable and solid, like we were meant to be for life. Those over-the-top, extravagant demonstrations of love were a regular occurrence in the early days and they won me over. I didn't know what I do now – that love is about consistency, stability, nurture and compassion, not about random and insincere declarations to total strangers.

Why did I fall for clients, you might ask? Quite simply, it was easier to date a client who already knew about my job than date someone who didn't, and risk being at the receiving end of shame and abuse when being open and honest with them. Believe it or not, sex workers believe in love too. Just a few months ago, I set up an account on the dating app Hinge. It was a stark reminder of why I dated clients in the past. My anxiety levels went through the roof when I locked in a couple of first dates. I decided I couldn't go through with them. What would I say when they asked what I did? If I wasn't honest and the date went well, I would be aware that I had lied to them from the off. If I was honest, I risked potential judgement, shaming, even being called a whore. Luckily, they did the job for me and cancelled on me anyway. I had never been so happy to be cancelled on and deleted my account soon after.

• • •

As our relationship progressed, cracks started to show, and I began to see certain sides to Shaun that I found very confusing. The warning signs were subtle – I was in love and the good was definitely outweighing the bad. So, like too many of us do, I tried not to pay them too much attention.

The first incident that I couldn't ignore came when I accidently knocked his drink over. He had left a glass of port on the floor next to the bed. As I was on the floor cleaning up, Shaun towered over me; his eyes glazed over and turned jet black. Through gritted teeth, he barked at me, 'You're pathetic!' I was shocked and didn't know what to think.

Shortly after this incident, I had a session with my therapist (as part of our master's in acting we were offered free therapy so I grabbed the opportunity) and told him what had happened. He responded, 'That is absolutely without a shadow of a doubt abusive behaviour.' This way of seeing his behaviour had never crossed my mind because the relationship had felt so idyllic. It was so confusing and I couldn't accept it. My therapist also advised that Shaun was displaying signs of narcissistic behaviour. I had no clue what that really meant. As far as I was aware, I had never come across a narcissist before. So, I decided to research it. As I began reading about the signs of narcissistic behaviour, I felt physically sick. Shaun ticked all the boxes. Fear and panic came over me. I had to get out of my flat and go for a walk around the Heath. This was not something that I was willing or ready to accept. By this time, I was head over in heels in love and ready to spend the rest of my life with Shaun. I couldn't imagine my life without him.

After about six months together, we both went to Bedfordshire for the weekend for the wedding of my school friend, Jessica. It was a long day, as weddings usually are, and I was exhausted afterwards. I just wanted to crash out at the hotel. I had previously promised Shaun a night of passion. Mistake. I passed out and woke up to an irate Shaun. He told me that something was wrong with me and that I should go and see a doctor about wanting to sleep all the time. I began to think that something *was* wrong with me. I did sometimes fall asleep early; just get me in a warm, dark room and I am catching flies within minutes. *Perhaps this isn't normal?* I thought. *Should I see a doctor?* His words hurt. Things had been so incredibly perfect and I loved floating around on cloud nine. I did not want to come back down to earth. The easiest way to deal with it was to wake up the next day and pretend it didn't happen.

This became a pattern. Shaun would often tell me that I 'wasn't right in the head' and that I needed to 'go and see someone'. Yet when I did start seeing my therapist again, he was convinced that I was fucking him, would give me the third degree and tell me that I couldn't see him anymore.

ELIZABETH G.

It was never his fault, always everybody else's. He could never turn inward and own up to anything. And yet he was Prince Charming to everybody else. In social situations he was the life and soul of the party – charismatic, energetic and vibrant, like the man I met the day I first walked through his door.

I began to learn about Shaun's past traumas. While spending the weekend together at my parents' farm, he opened up and told me about his father being murdered. He completely broke down. There it was right in front of me – all of his vulnerabilities laid bare. He was wailing in pain, like a scared little boy. At that point, I knew I had to support him and help him overcome his demons. He needed me. I wasn't going to be the woman who turned her back on him. I would be the woman who stood by him, loved and supported him.

After about eight months, Shaun persuaded me to move in with him. I was reluctant to give up my home in north London and move east, but we were so in love and I wanted to start building a life together. He had given up his home where we first met, to save money (or so I was told), and was temporarily living back with his mum. The plan was to start house hunting together and stay at his mum's in the short term to save money. Little did I know how rapidly things would change once we started living together.

As soon as I moved in, he had complete control over my movements. He started to control my finances, who I spent my time with, where I socialised. He slowly began to isolate me from my friends and family.

'Your family don't give a shit about you. It's time you face facts, your family don't want anything to do with you!'

'I can get girls like you 24/7.'

'I'm going to get myself a couple of nice Russian prostitutes.'

'You're a shit actor.' This one hurt the most, to the point where I was starting to believe him. Even though I had been signed with an agent and was starting to gain experience in fringe theatre and short films, I could feel my dream of becoming a professional actor in London slipping further and further away.

I now understand that his love bombing of me (for those not familiar with the term, this involves a continuous bombardment of love and affection that is relentless, convincing and not considerate of other people's boundaries) in the early part of our relationship was all part of the cycle of an abusive relationship; a tactic to lure the other person in. Because who in their right mind would hang around long enough to see how it all turns out if the abuser revealed their true self on the first date? Domestic violence involves a slow and calculated manipulation over a long period of time. By the time the abuse is in full swing, the person on the receiving end is so confused, longing for the charming Mr or Mrs Right to reappear and for things to go back to how they were in the beginning. Almost like taking that first drop of ecstasy, then constantly chasing that first high. It's never going to reappear again, but you live in the hope that one day it will.

He would call me obsessively, break things in front of me, display violence around me. On Valentine's Day he threatened to cut my hair off, and took off and left when I wouldn't open my legs wide enough for him to slide his fingers inside me when we were in a cab. He'd love bomb me one minute and disown me the next. He became very insistent on moving the relationship on very quickly and asked me to marry him after only a few months of dating. When things got really bad he would spit aggressively in my face while on top of me during sex and mock me for crying. I realised the mistake I'd made in allowing him to buy me a phone. The constant threats to cut it off were exhausting. *Why is he being like this?* I thought. *What happened to the lovable, vibrant, happy man I met? Why does he hate me so much?*

While listening to the radio one day, the topic of domestic violence came up. It literally stopped me in my tracks: 'He would control me with money and mock me for crying.' It was like a total stranger had just described my life. That's when I knew something was seriously wrong. Shaun had total control over me. In convincing me to move out of my home and leave my job, I had lost all financial independence and freedom to do what I wanted when I wanted. The free-spirited version of me was being crushed by a man so traumatised by his demons that he took it all out on me. On top of that, I was beginning to isolate from my friends and family. I was right where he wanted me.

I honestly thought that my life would be over if we broke up, that I'd have no friends, no social life, no money, nowhere to live. Because that's what perpetrators do. They slowly but surely make you feel totally worthless. They burrow that thought so deep into your head over a prolonged period of time, so convincingly, that you end up believing them. He had dehumanised me to the point where I felt good to nobody. I was beginning to give up on myself.

There were still good times in between, of course. Because abusive relationships still have happy times, believe it or not. Along with fear and isolation, this is what keeps the survivor in the relationship. Abusive behaviour operates in a cycle: tension, incident, reconciliation and honeymoon. And around the cycle goes, around and around like an insane merry-go-round on jet-fuelled steroids.

The 'honeymoon' phase and good times were what I clung to. We'd go out to clubs and parties. We had a great group of friends that we socialised with. That's really what our life together was all about: drugs and partying. I wanted to party at that point in my life and I especially loved the London nightlife scene. Shaun was a great energy to be around in that environment. We shared the same taste in dance music and loved being out with our friends dancing the night away. The dance floor was where we could both escape and feel free from past traumas. That's what we had in common: we were both numbing something from our past. It was just at home behind closed doors where the real issues in our relationship lay.

One night he grabbed me by the throat, clamping his hand tight and restricting my airway, and ordered me to go upstairs into the bedroom. He was full of rage after a disagreement about something trivial, yet again. At first I refused but it only added fuel to the fire, and I was scared what his next move would be if I didn't follow orders. Shaun was a big guy with broad shoulders and strong arms. Once that glaze came over his eyes and all I could see was darkness, the saliva yet again propelling through his teeth like venom, he was not someone that I wanted to challenge. During another argument, he raised his fist to me as if he was going to punch me.

'Go on then,' I said out of complete exhaustion. 'You'd be doing me a favour.' He pulled away.

All in all, I lasted just a few weeks in Ilford before I fled. My intuition got me out of there. I packed up a small bag of my things, put a plan in place and, while he was out, made a run for it. I had made arrangements to stay at a friend's house. This became a running theme over the next few months; spare rooms, spare beds, sofa surfing, sleeping on floors. Anywhere that was away from Shaun. I was going from place to place for months with no fixed address. I was in survival mode. I managed to get work temping in an office, which felt like a welcome relief. Returning to sex work never even crossed my mind at that point. I was too terrified that if Shaun found out he would follow through with his threat to kill me. In yet another power grab, he had threatened to 'out' me as a sex worker to my parents many times.

I soon began running out of options. I was down to my last £100. I decided to call a women's refuge shelter to see if they had any spare beds but unfortunately, because I wasn't a single mother or disabled, they could not accept me. As I sat in the pub next to work, nowhere to go, panic started to set in. I contemplated sleeping out on the Heath as it was a place I knew well, but something stopped me. I decided to use my last £100 on a room for the night in a Travelodge at King's Cross. I hadn't washed my clothes for some time and managed to wash everything in the bathtub, but by morning they were still damp and I ended up carrying a bag of soggy clothes to work the next day. I must have looked so spaced out sitting at my desk. I really don't know how I managed to get any work done and hold that job down. I would sit in the toilets and cry at least a few times a day. I could not believe that my life had come to this.

The next day, I swallowed my pride, called my mum and told her everything that had been going on. As soon as I had finished work that day, I was on a train home. I stayed on the farm for a few days and got some much-needed rest. I returned to London with a fresh mindset and feeling a little stronger. I made arrangements to stay with some of my fellow students from acting school. They gave up their lounge and sofa for me for a small sum of rent. I was truly grateful for their generosity.

Even though I blocked his number, Shaun still found a way to get through to me. He would call from a withheld number obsessively, leave voicemail after voicemail. It was exhausting. He wore me down and eventually I agreed to meet up with him. This just started another cycle. We'd meet up, try to work things out, get on, then fall out. Shaun would harass me, begging me to go back to him, declaring his undying love for me while crying down the phone, seemingly a broken man. This was then later followed by endless threats. He would threaten to kill me, himself or any potential boyfriends I dare meet.

Coming to terms with the fact that I was in an abusive relationship was one of the hardest things I have ever had to face. I hated the word 'victim'. I didn't want to think of myself as a victim. I didn't want pity or sympathy, I just wanted to not be living in the nightmare. Every time I called the National Domestic Abuse Helpline, the lines would always be busy. I would often find myself looking out of the window and thinking of the hundreds if not thousands of other people out there who were also experiencing domestic violence. What were they going through? Did they feel scared and alone like me? Where were they? Next door? At the end of the street? Did they feel suicidal too?

I was still auditioning. I hadn't totally given up on my acting. During one of my one-on-one singing lessons while preparing for a panto audition, my teacher and I were trying to play a recording through my phone but couldn't because of Shaun's obsessive calling. He must have tried about fourteen times. 'Tell him to fuck off!' my usually conservative teacher said. He was totally shocked. And it was shocking for me to see my teacher's reaction. I realised that I had become so used to his behaviour that I no longer thought of it as unusual. I simply expected it. I needed to see the shock again.

Then one good thing happened – somehow I got the panto job. I was absolutely ecstatic and could not wait to get on the road and begin touring. It was good to be out of London, to be working, to take my mind off things. But all my problems were still waiting for me. After the tour finished, I hit rock bottom. I was living with my good friend Maria who had been kind enough to open up her spare room to me. However, I now had no job, no money, no relationship, and I still had bills and rent to pay.

During this time, there was one person who slowly helped me to fight my way back. Who spoke to me on a daily basis and helped me to see that my life wasn't completely over because of one abusive man. She encouraged me to return to the land of the living when all I wanted to do was hide away and die. It was my mum. We had never been super close and rarely saw eye to eye. I was always the positive one, seeing the good in everything and everyone, and her negativity and constant worrying would always grind on me. But none of that mattered. She was my strength at a time when I felt so weak. I will never forget her love and encouragement at a time when I had totally given up on myself. Thanks, Mum, for your support.

'Just have a walk around the local pubs and bars and ask if they are looking for bar staff,' she said in the most understanding and encouraging way. 'Yep, OK, Mum,' I said. Bar work was the last thing I wanted to do but I knew that I had to find something, anything, to get me out of this hole. So, I did exactly what my mum advised. I got out of the house and spent the afternoon walking around Putney and asked around all the pubs, bars and restaurants. Anywhere and everywhere. Within a few days I had a trial at a local bar. The trial went well and the following week I had weekend shifts booked in. It was only temporary, I had to keep telling myself. I didn't particularly enjoy it but it was great to be out in a sociable environment earning money. Even talking to guys again was a real confidence boost. I couldn't believe it when a guy would start flirting with me and asked if I had a boyfriend.

While living with Maria in Putney, I discovered the Women's Aid Survivors' Forum. I was shocked to see so many stories similar to my own. Women who were suicidal, had nightmares, kept going back and finding it hard to move on. I couldn't believe it: there were many more women out there with so many stories of abuse to tell, all asking for help and supporting each other. I felt compelled to respond and support other abuse victims. In helping others, I began to realise my own strength. We helped to heal each other.

• • •

ELIZABETH G.

I never knew that the aftermath of leaving an abuser would be just as traumatising, if not more so, than staying. The nightmares, fears, anxiety, depression, PTSD. I lived in constant fear of wetting myself. I had to resort to wearing sanitary pads every day for the best part of a year. I began to hate the night; it terrified me. The bold and courageous Elizabeth was now a fearful little mouse scared of her own shadow. The psychological damage from his abuse was hard to escape. I feared it was something that would never leave me. I just could not get him out of my head. Even at night he was there, terrorising my dreams. I had nightmares of him raping me, chasing after me and trying to kill me. 'Stupid fucking cunt!' he'd once shouted. 'The only thing you are good for is doing a job that involves opening your legs!' I couldn't stop replaying the abuse in my mind.

Then came the tears. I cried and cried and cried. I never knew it was possible to produce so many tears. I felt deeply sad. I still loved him very much and missed him more than I had ever missed anyone. 'How can you miss and love someone who treated you so badly?' many people asked. As awful as he was to me, there were good times, and the good times were some of the happiest moments of my life. He made me feel incredibly special and loved, like the most adored and protected woman in the world. That was what I was holding on to. It became a constant internal battle between the love I had for him and the disgusting way he treated me.

After the tears came the anger. I was furious at him for putting me in this situation. I remember so clearly that when we first met, I wasn't hugely attracted to him; I could have happily continued with my life without him pursuing me. But no, he lured me in of course. Most of all, I was angry at myself. How could I have been so stupid to fall for a man's charm? My insecurities and reliance on men to make me feel good about myself had put me in this position and I only had myself to blame.

Of course, it wasn't until I started reading about and researching abusive partners and relationships that I realised that actually, there was nothing I could have done. I was not to blame. Shaun knew exactly what he was doing to me from the moment he laid eyes on me, and I fell victim to him from the moment I walked through his door. One of the most valuable lessons I took from this experience was to rely on no one but myself to make me feel good. Seeking gratification and approval from others was my absolute curse and I resolved never to rely on a man's flattering words to make me feel special ever again.

I slowly started to get my social life back. While getting myself ready, I could once again take my time without someone screaming and shouting at me for taking too long. I had forgotten what it felt like to be able to just take my time without someone breathing down my neck and giving me a hard time about it every two seconds. Fast forward to today, and being rushed by someone is still an absolute trigger. It sends me into total panic. Sorry for snapping at you when you asked me if I had booked the Uber, Mum. It was just a trigger.

I finally found the courage to go to the police and told them everything. It was such a release, and my way of taking back some control of my life. They were unable to take any action due to a lack of evidence but at least they were informed, the events had been recorded and I received a crime number. It was a big first step. I was advised on the difficulty of proving incidents of domestic violence.

The police officer was incredibly understanding; I even told him how we met. The officer was not at all surprised that Shaun had used this as a way to control me. To Shaun, I was an easy target because I was a sex worker; he used shame and stigma as leverage.

And I did feel shame. I lived with a constant cloak of it hanging over me. With Shaun's aid, I convinced myself that I was just a bad person who did not deserve happiness. I was tormented by anxiety and lived in total fear of Shaun following through with his threat to drive to my parents' house and tell them that I was a sex worker. There needs to be laws and regulations against this type of behaviour. It's time for the bullies and the cowards to stop threatening sex workers into a corner of shame. The louder and prouder we are, the less power we give to people like Shaun.

•••

After almost a year of moving from place and place and working towards gaining the strength to move on with my life, I moved back in with Shaun. Yes, I hear you. I understand what you are thinking. Why the hell did I put myself back in that situation? There are many reasons. The one most obvious to survivors but baffling to outsiders was quite simply, it felt safer. His threats to kill me felt very real.

I had done the research. I knew the statistics. I didn't want to become one of them.

He became his most volatile and threatening when I told him I was moving on. He had nothing to lose. The threats would terrify me to the point where I became an emotional wreck. At least having him in my life and being more amicable made his erratic behaviour a lot easier to predict. It was the silences and not knowing what his next move would be that really scared me. I was reading a lot about abusive behaviour and believed this was enough armour against him. *Crazy Love* by Leslie Morgan Steiner and *Why Does He Do That? Inside the Minds of Angry and Controlling Men* by Lundy Bancroft helped me to rebuild my strength and understand the patterns of his behaviour better. Reading empowered me.

In addition to this, the natural empath in me couldn't refuse to see him. He would still cry down the phone to me like a little boy, begging to see me. He told me he was going to kill himself if I didn't. He was so convincing. I believed him. I told him I was seeing someone else and he sounded truly heartbroken. I have never heard a grown man cry like that before, sobbing his heart out, barely able to catch his breath. Despite everything, I hated the fact that I had hurt him so much by telling him the truth. He asked me to stop seeing him but I refused. But his harassing me and begging me became exhausting. Some days it just felt easier to give in and say yes. He was overwhelmingly powerful in his conviction that we should be together and there were times when I felt too weak to fight it. It was then that he was able to swoop in and lure me back.

The first couple of months of living together again were idyllic. Shaun was having regular therapy sessions, which were proving to be incredibly effective. We had given the party lifestyle the boot; he was off the cocaine and we were focused on a healthy and happy future together. The change in his personality was huge; with the help of a therapist and the elimination of drugs, he was the kindest and most lovable man. He was finally tackling his demons from the past; I could see a really positive change in him and was so incredibly proud. I fell in love with him all over again.

However, as time progressed the cracks began to show yet again, but they became even darker and deeper than before. Things soon spiralled and became the worst they had ever been. I was so angry at myself for believing his lies all over again. I felt like I was constantly screaming on the inside. I stopped calling my friends and family and once again became isolated from the rest of the world. I was like a walking zombie, dead inside.

It was frustrating but not one bit surprising. The only positive that I had to hold on to was that I had been here before and managed to get out; I had previously lost my sense of self and yet regained my strength, my power and the essence of who I was. I knew I would have to fight to get it all back.

I was already working a new job by the time I moved back in with Shaun so at least I had that going for me. It was a job that I loved and took to very well. I was working as a qualified massage therapist. Just massage this time. No happy endings. That job became a game changer. It was good money and I was working with a fabulous group of ladies. Among the team were many fellow creatives and actors. So not only did it become my financial stability, it also became my social life away from Shaun.

After around three months of living back together, I took a trip home to Bedfordshire to see my friends from school just for the day. I was so excited. It was the first time I was to spend time with my friends since I'd got back with Shaun. The day before, I spent hours in Mothercare buying gifts for their little ones. I hardly ever saw them, and it meant so much to me. I wanted to spoil them rotten!

As I made my way back to London, Shaun was constantly calling me and texting me saying he was worrying about me. I felt my stomach tie in knots as I tried to convince him time and time again that I was fine and on the way back. I got frustrated and shouted at him to stop worrying about me; it felt like I was being suffocated. Big mistake. An argument erupted and regrettably I called him a prick. Boy, did I pay for that mistake.

Shaun was waiting for me at the station. I got in the car hoping we'd managed to resolve things on the phone. I was wrong. Yet another screaming match erupted. He punched the steering wheel so hard that he bent it. 'That's it, I've had it, I'm going to crash this fucking car!' he exclaimed. The rage was pumping through his veins like a man possessed. His eyes were fierce and filled with hate. I had my head down. I was terrified and quivering all over, bracing myself for the impact of the crash. He began speeding up and braking erratically. I began to fear for my life. *Shit, shit, I am going to die. I'm so scared – he is acting crazy – he is actually going to crash the car. Please, God, please make him stop. I just want to get out of this car!* I wondered how I would be injured. *Will the impact knock me out? Will the car burst into flames? Will I burn to death? Will my bones break? Will I be crushed? What if we kill other motorists on the road? Will I end up disfigured? Oh God, oh God, I need to get out of this car!*

I was hysterical and begging him not to crash the car. 'Please don't do this, please don't crash the car. Please, Shaun, I love you so much! Just please slow down!' I pleaded as I sobbed and sobbed my broken heart out. It made no difference. If anything, it made him worse. He continued to speed down the motorway like a crazed animal. The sounds that came out of him were not those of a human.

That journey along the motorway felt like the longest of my life. I felt overwhelmed with relief when we were finally off and at the roundabout close to his house. Whatever the reason – perhaps I had a guardian angel watching over me that night – he did not crash the car and for that, at least, I was thankful. The worst of the storm apparently over, he pulled over to get a takeaway. As soon as the car stopped, I was out of the door and making a run for it.

I had no idea where I was going or what to do. I was terrified. All I knew was that I had to be as far away from him as possible, even if that meant sleeping rough for the night. It was safer than being around him. I could hear him shouting at me but I kept running, allowing my instinct to take the lead. He got back in his car and caught up with me. He jumped out and grabbed me by my arm. I pulled away. 'Get off me!' I cried.

'Get your arse in that car now!'

'No!' I said. There was no way I was getting back in that car anytime soon after the journey through hell. 'I'll come back to the takeaway but by foot. I will come back, but there is no way I am going in the car with you.' He accepted my offer, and we met back at the takeaway.

We both sat in the car (engine off, doors open at my insistence), his tone completely changed. 'I'm sorry for scaring you,' he sobbed.

'It's OK,' I said. I hated to see him upset; it broke my heart.

I was so angry at myself that I had let this person back into my life. I knew the facts and statistics when it came to abusive relationships – I'd spent enough nights researching the subject. I knew about the manipulation of the 'victim' by the perpetrator. No matter what he said, I reminded myself that it was just another tactic, doing everything I could to make sure that I didn't get sucked into his 'I love you, baby, I want to see you.' And yet here I was again.

He was acting the same way he used to when he'd taken cocaine, and sure enough, when I confronted him about it he reacted just as he used to when he was lying to me constantly. 'No, I haven't been on the fucking gear, you aggravating pest!' Why oh why was he acting like this again? Was it drugs? Was it because his therapist was away and he hadn't seen her for a few weeks? I just wanted the truth.

As angry and unpredictable as he was, this time I wasn't going to back down. I began fighting back. 'I'm just asking you not to make nasty comments like that. It's not nice. I have booked a session with my therapist for next Monday. You need to go and see your therapist too,' I said, hoping that this would help him to regain a little clarity on the situation, but it didn't work.

'You do not tell me what I can and can't say! Who the fuck do you think you are?'

We were having this argument in a car park. I got out of the car and headed straight to the toilets. I had to get away from him. I could hear him shouting obscenities behind me but still I carried on walking and two men in a Range Rover stopped abruptly and asked me if I was OK. They looked shocked. I just nodded, half smiled and continued. That was a real moment. In another life, I would have said, 'No, I'm not OK at all, can I come with you?' But I just didn't want to risk getting others involved for fear of what Shaun might do to them. In choosing to walk away, I was protecting them. But even to this day, I always remember that moment so clearly. That's when I knew that something was very, very wrong, when total strangers tried to offer help and came up to me to ask if I was OK. I can still see the look on their faces as they sat in their car watching and observing in disbelief. They weren't the first brave souls who tried to intervene. There was another car park incident when a kind man stepped in, only to receive a barrage of abuse as Shaun diverted his anger towards him. To all the brave people who tried to help, I am so grateful to you and have never forgotten your kindness at a time when I needed it the most.

When Shaun finally convinced me to get back in the car, it was once again the journey from hell. He continued with his screaming and shouting, punching the steering wheel, shouting 'cunt' to anyone and everyone that got in his way until we arrived back in sunny Ilford.

I went straight upstairs. I was exhausted and desperately wanted to get some sleep. I lay on the bed and he entered the room.

I felt the intensity of his energy and it was evident that he was going to hold on to this argument for as long as he could. A switch had been flicked and there was nothing I could do about it. I felt as if I was sinking.

The argument escalated further: something in him had been triggered and I was going to bear the brunt of it. I just wanted it to end. 'Can you please just let me get some sleep?' I said, keeping my composure in the hope that things would dwindle and he would forget about it. As the argument worsened, I moved to the edge of the bed; it was the furthest I could get away from him in that tiny little room. In his fit of rage he leant over and hit my leg. He was out of control. It wasn't painful, just a mediocre smack over the thigh. Just enough to intimidate me and make me feel completely worthless.

'Ouch, don't hit me!' I said.

'Sorry, I'm sorry! Come here, I'm really sorry.' I couldn't believe how quickly his tone changed.

He somehow then managed to escalate the argument again by telling me I needed to go and see my therapist, implying that something was wrong with me. I was furious that he would continue to suggest this after what he had just done. I started packing. He grabbed all my stuff and threw it around the room. Then he took my suitcase and threw it at me. He grabbed me with one hand either side of my mouth, pulling me up by my face from the ground. His hands were tight around my face like a clamp that would not release. When he finally let go, I felt as though I had been punched. I was worried I would have bruises on my face and would have to cover them up for work. When I checked the next day, there were no bruises; as usual, he was too clever to be that careless and leave physical proof. Shortly after he began trying it on with me. How the hell was he in the mood for sex after that fight? Did being aggressive towards me turn him on?

Another day, Shaun returned home early one morning after working a night shift. He entered the bedroom like an animal possessed. Something about his energy told me that I needed to be on guard more than ever. An argument erupted when I tried closing the window. That's all it took. He was just waiting for the opportunity to make his move.

He started calling me a paranoid schizophrenic and yet again told me that I 'wasn't right in the head'. I challenged him and he spat in my face. He then pulled his shoulders back and looked as though he was about to head butt me. I braced myself for the impact. But then something stopped him and he stuck his finger in my mouth instead. Not satisfied with leaving it at that, he then hit me on my back and arm a few times after I tried pushing him off. He proceeded to clamp his hands on either side of my cheeks and squeezed so hard that, yet again, I felt like I had been punched in the face. Things then began to really spiral to the point where they were the worst they had ever felt. His eyes burned with a total hatred for me. He kicked me, shoved me, intimidated me and punched me in the head multiple times. He hit me with his clothing, pulled the duvet over my head and proceeded to call me a 'whore, a bitch and a cunt'. I longed for peace.

He threw me onto the bed when I tried again to close the window. I didn't want the neighbours hearing. He straddled over me and put his hand in position ready to strangle me. I mentally prepared myself. Again, something stopped him and instead he bit my ear. 'Get off me!' I screamed. I managed to push him off. I asked him to just stop being nasty and let me go to sleep but he couldn't leave it; he was restless and aggressive and nothing

I did was going to calm him down. I tried calling my mum, but she didn't answer so I left a voicemail. This infuriated him, so he grabbed my phone and demanded to know who it was. 'Was that your boyfriend, was it? You can get your stuff and you can fuck off! I want you gone!'

I tried my hardest not to get upset or show any kind of emotion. I didn't want him to see that he was getting to me. 'That's fine,' I said. 'It's all been arranged.'

His response made him sound more crazy than ever. 'Oh, it's been arraaaaanged! Fucking ponce!'

It made my skin crawl. He had completely and utterly lost the plot, it seemed to me. It was a moment of total madness where he had lost all awareness of himself and his surroundings.

In that moment, I remembered what the police had advised me about domestic violence being hard to prove. I wanted to get that evidence. For myself more than anything. So that nobody could discredit me or accuse me of making up lies. He was always too smart (like a lot of abusers) to do so much damage that he would leave physical marks on me, which is why I knew I had to record the abuse on my phone.

I positioned my phone under my pillow and turned the audio recorder on. I was terrified that he'd find out and smash up my phone like he had done to his own phone so many times in the past. But I just knew I had to take that risk. I was following my gut and instinct took over. I did something that was incredibly brave but at the same time I did not really think through the consequences if he found out. Luckily, he did not.

The fact that I had told him I had made arrangements to leave but he had no clue where I was going infuriated him. The truth was, I had no idea where I was going myself; I was bluffing. All I knew was that I had to get out of that dangerous and unpredictable situation. In his fit of rage he believed me.

To my great relief, he began to gather his things. He decided he was going out to play golf. As he left the bedroom, he turned to me and barked at me one last time: 'Cunt!' It poured through his gritted teeth like venom. He said exactly what he thought of me and he meant it.

As soon as he left, I went into full survival mode. I spoke to my parents and arranged for them to come and pick me up. They weren't surprised; were probably almost relieved that I was finally fleeing. They didn't question it. They dropped everything to come and get me. That, right there, that one act of dropping everything without question in order to get me out of a dangerous situation, that is love. I've never forgotten it.

I began packing. My focus was on getting the hell out of there as quickly and as safely as I could. I was convinced that if I stayed, he would kill me. His look of hatred and disdain towards me that morning told me everything I needed to know and was my motivation to get out of there. A number of times I thought about calling the police but I didn't want to aggravate him further. I was terrified of what his response would be. It was all fear.

We were still living with his mum. She had been home that morning and would have heard everything. As she would have done on many other occasions. She never intervened. I told her what had happened. By then I was a broken mess and didn't have the strength to hide it. 'Oh,' she said after I explained to her that her son had just bitten me on the ear, kicked me and crushed my face in his hands. I don't resent her for it. Looking back, I think she was just as scared of him as I was but loved him all the same. As did I for so long. She was a kind-hearted person and always made me feel welcome. Even though she never intervened, I was still grateful to her.

My mum and dad just got in the car and drove to Ilford. They brought the dog with them too. I didn't want them at Shaun's house. I didn't want there to be a confrontation if he suddenly showed up and risk them getting hurt. So I arranged for us to meet at the station. I loaded all my possessions into an Uber as quickly as I could. The driver started to complain about all my belongings but then he noticed the look of total panic and fear on my face. His tone quickly changed and he became patient and understanding. Luckily Shaun did not come home, and we sped out of there.

I greeted my parents with hugs and tears, and we transferred my belongings from the Uber into their car. I thanked the driver profusely for his kindness. He pointed to the sky and assured me that everything would work out and that this was all part of life's plan. All loaded up, strapped in and with the dog on my lap for comfort, we began our journey home. '(Something Inside) So Strong' started playing on the radio. *Of all the songs*, I thought. I held the dog for some much-needed reassurance while she licked the tears that were streaming down my face (dogs just know). As we began our journey home, I gazed out of the window a broken woman. I was emotionally drained, exhausted, battered and feeling totally defeated. I longed for peace, for rest and a good night's sleep.

• • •

Shit things happen and I'm not one to give a sob story. Playing the victim is beneficial to no one. And anyway, I hate the word 'victim' – I am a survivor. I don't believe that we are defined by the things that happen *to* us – it's about how we choose to deal with them. And it really is a choice. We can wallow in self-pity and adopt a victim mentality, or we can choose to rise above it and use the experiences to help us strengthen and grow. The experience with Shaun is a crucial part of my story. I learnt so many life lessons from it. I took something that was really shit and learnt how to use it to my advantage. Realising my inner strength after being tested by adversity made me bulletproof.

Domestic violence knows no boundaries. It does not just happen to one age group, race, gender, profession or social class. Domestic violence can affect anyone and everyone. Back then, I didn't know how to implement healthy boundaries or prioritise my own needs in relationships. It was all about their needs and putting them first.

I was never one to take heartache well. I am a sensitive soul. I feel things very deeply. In some ways, it's a wonderful quality to have, to feel things deeply, to have an awareness of myself and others. I have been told numerous times over the years, 'You are too sensitive.' It's exactly what Shaun and the bullies have said. There is no such thing as being too sensitive in my view. It's what you do with that sensitivity that matters.

Contrary to what some people might assume, the biggest danger for me while working as a sex worker came from matters of the heart. It was falling in love with clients that got me into the worst situations. I look back and cringe at how vulnerable I made myself. Threats to 'out' us can really panic sex workers and leave us in a distressed and isolated state. It is never anybody else's place to out a sex worker. Telling others is our decision and our decision alone. There really needs to be clear laws against this type of behaviour.

My experiences are a prime example of what shame can do. I felt ashamed of being in an abusive relationship. Of returning to a man only for him to abuse me all over again. Shame caused me to hide my abusive relationship and make out like everything was OK. Added to this was the shame I felt about being a sex worker and the fear of people in my life finding out. It caused me to isolate and shut down. Shame made me vulnerable. It empowered others to hold their knowledge of my job over me, to abuse me and keep me silent.

While I was writing this chapter, the legendary Tina Turner passed away. I found it strange to sob so hysterically over a person I had never met. But I felt deeply connected to her. She was the original girl power. We were both survivors of domestic violence. Reading about her story strengthened me and gave me hope. It showed me that there was light at the end of a very long tunnel. That I would come out of this experience a stronger person. She left Ike with practically nothing but her stage name. She cleaned and scrubbed toilets to survive. She remained focused on her goals, she never gave up, she persisted through the tough times while working hard to make a name for herself as a solo artist, becoming a hugely successful singer in her forties.

In the weeks before her death, she said she wanted to be remembered 'as the Queen of Rock 'n' Roll. As a woman who showed it's OK to strive for success on your own terms.' She is a true inspiration for anyone, particularly a survivor of domestic violence. Thank you, Tina, I am so grateful to you. A woman like no other.

CHAPTER SEVEN
AFTERMATH

'Guilty.'

There it was. The verdict I had been hoping for but dreaded may never come. The nightmare was finally over. The heaviness of the past few months was gone. Lifted. All the stress, the worry and the sleepless nights were finished. Justice had been served and I was able to finally start moving on with my life.

The day of Shaun's trial was like nothing I had ever experienced before, nor do I ever want to experience it again. The thought of having to face my abusive ex in court filled me with fear but it was something that I just knew I had to do. This wasn't all about me. It was also to prevent him from abusing others. I wasn't standing up just for myself that day, but for all victims and survivors of domestic violence. The Metropolitan Police and Witness Support had been incredible throughout the whole process. I was even able to go and view the courtroom pre-trial, which really helped to take away a lot of the anxiety I was feeling in the build-up.

I was adamant that I had to have a screen that would prevent me from being able to see Shaun and from Shaun being able to see me. I was still very much in fear of wetting myself at the time and so also requested to sit while giving evidence rather than stand. These requests were granted.

I attended court on my own. No support network, just myself. At the time, I was incredibly hurt that my family did not come to support me, to hold my hand and reassure me. But now, looking back, I am grateful that I went through that experience on my own. It taught me resilience. It also meant that while sitting in witness protection waiting to go through to the courtroom, I was able to zone out from all the chaos around me (and it was total chaos!). There was every kind of emotion imaginable in that room. I didn't allow any of it to affect me. It was a strange experience. It was almost as if I was tapping into a different part of my brain, mentally preparing myself for battle, but at the same time I felt calm and stable. Grounded.

I was on two types of medication at the time: propranolol and oxazepam. Propranolol was for the physical side of my panic attacks, helping to lower my heart rate. Oxazepam was to help with the mental side of my panic attacks, easing my mind so I wasn't in a state of constant high alert. At first I didn't want to take anything before the trial, but just before I left the house I decided not to risk it, not to be a hero. I had been having panic attacks left, right and centre; triggers were everywhere, from a car door slamming to shouting and any kind of loud noise, whether it be happy or sad.

I had been assured that the prosecutor was the best of the best. I found a moment to nervously explain to him that I was working as a sex worker when I first met Shaun. I was sure that the defence would use it as a way to discredit me. The prosecutor was incredibly supportive and reassuring. He explained that the magistrates were only interested in what happened on the day of the assault, not what I was doing for a living when I met Shaun.

When it was Shaun's turn to give evidence, I chose to leave the courtroom. I couldn't face listening to any more of his lies. I met with a fellow massage therapist in a coffee shop around the corner while awaiting the verdict. When the officer called and gave me the news, I looked at my colleague and burst into tears. I felt overwhelmed with relief. The war was over, and I could finally move on.

It was my therapist at the time who encouraged me to go to the police and report Shaun. 'He is never, ever going to leave you alone,' she said. The initial reaction from my local police station in my hometown totally undermined my experience. I was abruptly told that it 'will never go to court due to a lack of evidence'. *Good*, I thought. I didn't want to go to court or ever be in the same room as Shaun ever again. I just wanted him to leave me alone. For good. As the incident took place in London, it was a case for the Metropolitan Police. Luckily, they stepped up.

It was my therapist's words and also conversations with the National Domestic Abuse Helpline that gave me the strength to report him. I am hugely grateful to those important people. I was absolutely terrified but just knew that I had to do it for my own safety and for others he may abuse in the future. It started to feel like the only way out of the nightmare.

I became fascinated with the case of Hollie Gazzard and how the police had failed to protect her. Hollie did not have any physical scars. However, there were numerous signs that her ex had exhibited control over her. He began a campaign of harassment and then suddenly went quiet. The next day, he stabbed her fourteen times, killing her. It was when Shaun had gone quiet that I had been most scared, leading me to return to him time and time again. After hearing Hollie's story, I wanted to fight for what I believed in and ensure that the police did everything in their power to protect me.

Shaun received a fine – I think it was for £800 – was ordered to do community service and attend a 'Building Better Relationships' programme. A two-year restraining order was granted, which came as a welcome relief. On top of this, Shaun would have a criminal record for domestic violence. The fine and community service didn't mean much but the criminal record was what really mattered. Under Clare's Law, if anyone Shaun started dating in the future suspected that he had a history of domestic violence, they would be able to go to the police and have his name checked on a database where his record would be shown. A lifeline.

Living back home after I finally left Shaun was challenging. My family struggled to understand domestic violence, though Mum tried her best. I had lost all my independence – one of the most important things that made me, me – and on top of that I was a broken woman trying my hardest to focus on healing and moving on. It was easier said than done. Although not visible, the scars were clearly still there and were not going away anytime soon.

Being back on the farm, though not without its tensions, was a chance to heal, rest and catch up on some much-needed sleep. And, boy, did

I sleep. The endless stress of Shaun waking me up in the middle of the night after returning home from work was over. For that, at least, I was hugely thankful.

By the time the trial came, I was already living in a house share on the outskirts of London in Hertfordshire and working back as a massage therapist in London. I had grown to love this job and had missed it. Once the trial had finished, I put all my energy into rebuilding my life, moving on from Shaun and beginning the healing process.

• • •

One year on and I was healed enough to come off the meds and no longer felt constant, crippling anxiety. I wasn't scared of wetting myself anymore so could finally stop wearing sanitary pads every day and was still really enjoying my job, completing further massage training. Most importantly, I consciously appreciated and cherished my freedom every day. I was no longer living in fear.

In my journal, I wrote down some areas that I still wanted to work on. One was going to the gym more often and improving my fitness (some things never change!) and another was getting a better handle on my finances. I was working as a holistic massage therapist and it was my first real experience of being self-employed. Managing my accounts and doing tax returns was something that was all very alien and overwhelming to me.

I was also beginning to struggle month to month. Working as a massage therapist did not come with a guaranteed fixed income and my earnings were unpredictable. I had my first tax bill looming and I wasn't sure how I was going to pay it. I was so short of funds one weekend that I barely had enough money to get the train home for my dad's birthday. My dear friend Freddie, who I had stayed in touch with after acting school and who was one of the few people who had known about my life as a sex worker, was able to help me out and lend me money for my train ticket, but I felt so guilty having to ask for help.

As financial pressures began to mount, I once again debated going back to sex work. I felt nervous, but something was drawing me back. My focus was on my tax bill. I was losing sleep over how I would get it paid on time. I remember very clearly sitting on the backsteps of my London house share looking up to the sky and debating in my head the pros and cons of returning. It was never going to be a decision I would make lightly. I bit the bullet and called Lust. The only way I can explain it is as a strong, intuitive pull. It was my intuition that guided me back to the industry. *For whatever reason,* I thought, *I am meant to be in the adult industry.*

Kim remembered me straight away and my call was received with warmth. I felt relief that they welcomed me back with open arms. I soon began working at Lust as well as my massage job. I'd massage during the week and work at Lust on the weekends. It was the perfect balance. However, unable to afford to live on my own at that point, I was back to sneaking around. On the occasions I did a night shift at Lust on a weekday, I would have to hang out in McDonald's for a couple of hours until my housemates left for work so they wouldn't see me crawling into bed looking worse for wear. As with the house share when I was at acting school, this was a fine example of the stigma of being a sex worker. My new housemates – two guys, one girl, all postgrads – were much younger than me. Despite feeling unable to risk telling them the truth about my work, I did have a lot of fun times with them. I will always remember that house as the place where I began to rebuild my life post domestic violence.

In spite of the sneaking around, for the first time in a long time, I was starting to feel happy again. It might sound flippant but I've always said that working as a sex worker is the best way to get over a break-up. Getting dressed up, showered with compliments and being paid thousands of pounds to socialise and have sex was just the ego boost I needed after Shaun. Yet again, I was beginning to build a great list of like-minded clients who doted on me, and helped me to rebuild my confidence – as well as my finances. My earnings were soon increasing and the financial pressures lifted. I had two income streams. This is something that I still believe in today. Relying on one income stream, no matter what it was, always seemed like far too much pressure for me.

This was the point at which I really began to turn things around. All my focus was on working my way up in the adult industry, increasing my earnings and investing. I didn't know exactly how or in what at that stage, but my mind was starting to think bigger. I was determined to start setting myself up for the rest of my life so that I'd never have to rely on a man financially ever again. I had learnt the hard way what being financially dependent on a partner could mean. I may have had a way to go in my education where understanding money was concerned, but financial independence was, for the first time, at the forefront of my mind.

• • •

At Lust, bookings were just as varied as they had ever been. Maybe more so. Clients' ages ranged from the twenties up to the sixties; there was a lot of variation in social class and professions. I still did party bookings that would go on all through the night. I found I still wanted to party. Maybe it was partly the joy of simply surviving what I had been through, maybe it was a coping mechanism. But either way, the hedonist in me was still alive and well. I was getting more and more party bookings with fellow sex workers that I clicked with. At that time, I felt like I was living a dream. I was getting paid to party.

We travelled to some beautiful locations and stunning mansions, from Essex to north London, Buckinghamshire to Surrey. I was gaining momentum and building up a good list of regulars. Visiting a client that I already knew and got on well with was always my preference over meeting someone new. A huge part of the job of a sex worker – our key skill, if you like – is being able to make an immediate connection. To seemingly and effortlessly make an intimate situation with a stranger feel natural. I am proud of my ability to do this but it was still a relief to see my regulars and not to have to start from scratch with new people. Being back at Lust also meant I was able to see some of my favourite clients that I had not seen for years – like William and Mr Sassy.

One Friday evening, I received a request to visit a couple. I gladly accepted. Bookings with couples always excited me. Perhaps there was some assurance in a woman's presence. I entered the bedroom and saw two large plastic boxes. One was filled with clean dildos and the other was empty, for used ones, apparently. The man proceeded to explain that he enjoyed being fucked up the arse by a sex worker and his girlfriend enjoyed watching. It was a party booking so cocaine was free flowing. It was my first real taste of using a strap-on on a man and it intrigued me. I felt a strange sense of empowerment. They clearly had done this many times before. They had a very organised system as we transferred one dildo after the next into the 'used' box and watched it fill up as the night progressed.

During my time at Lust, I gained a lot of experience working with couples. I had the pleasure of visiting a super-sexy couple who had been up all night partying out in the suburbs. It was Sunday morning when they booked me. I was their last port of call before crashing out. After a brief chat and breaking the ice, the girlfriend leant over and began a slow and sensual kiss. We started to undress each other as the boyfriend watched.

As I lay back on the sofa with my legs wide open, the girlfriend lay on her front, put her head between my legs and slowly began to arouse my clitoris with her tongue. It was one of the first real sexual experiences I had with a woman. So far, it had been mostly kissing and licking nipples; this felt a lot more sensual, a lot more intimate. I was totally aroused. She continued to manoeuvre her tongue around my clitoris as I felt myself getting wetter and wetter. My clitoris began throbbing as I came closer to orgasm. Even today, ten years on, that moment is still one of my 'go to' memories for the wank bank.

I became aware that her boyfriend was hovering around my head, excitedly watching like a kid in a candy store, eagerly waiting for me to suck his cock. I could see it waving around from the corner of my eye. But I was so in the moment with his girlfriend that having his penis in my mouth felt like a nuisance at that point. We made our way into the bedroom. The girlfriend instructed me to straddle her boyfriend and ride him while she watched. 'Cum!' she kept saying to her boyfriend while looking at me, smiling from ear to ear.

However, there were some bookings with couples that did not go so well. Another couple I went to visit had also been partying through the weekend. Booking a sex worker was clearly the man's idea. Halfway through the booking, the girlfriend began to get jealous. I went into the bathroom to give them a moment and they started arguing. It's one of the most awkward situations for a sex worker to be in. I didn't want to stay but they had booked me for a certain amount of time so technically I was expected to stay there for the remainder of the booking. When I came out of the bathroom, they said everything was OK, but the atmosphere felt slightly hostile. I was still learning back then. If that happened today, I would have refunded some of the money and bolted out of the door. But I honoured the booking, stayed the remainder of my time and made a swift exit as soon as it was time to leave.

I have enjoyed having sex with women just as much as I have enjoyed having sex with men. It all comes down to chemistry. I have found that with women more often than not it is more sensual and less driven by ego. Which is not going to be the same for everyone obviously – that's just my observation over the years. Personally, I don't care about how many times and going all through the night, which usually happens only when cocaine is involved anyway, and more often than not results in 'limp cocaine dick' if Viagra is not present.

In my experience, women seem to have a better understanding of what it takes to make each other cum. That's not to say that men don't – I've met some men with the most incredible oral skills that have left my body pulsating for minutes afterwards. I can't speak for every woman, but personally, what it takes for me to cum is patience and consistency. No shouting orders or demands to cum. My vagina immediately closes up on orders to have an orgasm in order to satisfy a man's ego. Being sensual, gentle, the lightest touch, teasing the crap out of me, no shaking their head around all over the place and certainly no slapping my vulva. That is not pleasurable and does not help me – or many women, I don't think – to achieve orgasm. Keep the tongue on the target, eye on the prize, no diverting. Be patient and the fireworks will come. When I cum, you will know about it.

• • •

One of my favourite clients was a lovely man in his sixties who was retired. He was totally charming and lived alone. Without fail, he'd always have a cream cake and cup of tea waiting for me. He knew the way to my heart. Clients like this went straight to the top of my favourites list. We'd start the booking by catching up and having a good chat before fun and games in the bedroom. He'd often give me advice on managing my accounts and tax returns.

This client said something to me that has stuck with me all these years: 'I'm not paying you to stay, I'm paying you to leave.' Suddenly it became so crystal clear, so obvious. For so many, when they book a sex worker, the attraction is that once the experience has finished, at the end of the allotted time, that's it. Neither party has an obligation to the other. It was to the point and served its purpose in that moment without complications between two consenting adults. We'd have fun together, then be free to carry on living our lives.

Some bookings would have me travelling way out into the sticks. A regular client of the agency, though not someone I'd met before, requested a booking with me. When we arrived, we drove down a long and winding immaculate driveway. I was delighted to see that the client lived on a stud farm! Horses were grazing in the paddocks all around us. It felt like a home from home. Like I was able to reconnect with my country roots, even if just for a couple of hours.

I found myself visiting a number of older men living on their own in big houses, some of them widowers. The thing about loneliness is that it's a killer, literally. Experts say that lonely people are far more likely to die prematurely than those with healthy social relationships.[5] There are several reasons why loneliness can be deadly, and many ways in which feeling isolated can ruin lives. So, to those who struggle to understand and accept the profession of a sex worker, I ask them to consider all the people who are alone. Particularly older people. Not all of them can afford to pay for a sex worker. Not all of them would want to, of course. But for those who do, who do feel a need for intimate human contact, what would you suggest? Join a club? Volunteer? Hope to meet someone? Remain lonely if they don't?

• • •

Just like with my massage job, I learnt to accept that not every shift would be busy. One minute you are flavour of the month, the next minute: tumbleweed. I was grateful when work was busy but also came to understand that, at some point, chances are a dry spell will come. Of course, there are ways to help increase booking levels by adding selfies to online profiles and by updating professional photos every six months. Not always a guarantee but it can help. Nowadays, I find it so ironic that when I have bags of energy ready for a busy shift, feeling my healthiest and most refreshed and raring to go, there will be nothing. Yet on days when I am tired and in need of a break, bookings go through the roof. So, I've learnt to push through as much as my body can take. It's totally unpredictable. Sometimes there is just something in the air. Experience taught me to put money aside and nest rather than just blow it all when work was busy. Because at some point, those reserves will come in handy for the tumbleweed days.

One positive of quiet days at Lust was an opportunity to bond with the other ladies. During one of the summer heatwaves, work went totally dead so a couple of us opted to sunbathe on the rooftop of the office instead. Moments like that really connected us. It was important to have friends in the industry. However, while I have worked with so many lovely ladies over the years who have taught me a lot, there are always going to be colleagues you don't get on with. That's just life.

One day, I had to report a couple of the ladies, Kitty and Rachel, to the office manager. The three of us had been booked together for a party with a group of guys. Even before we arrived at the door, both ladies had a bad attitude, moaning about clients and the agency and projecting very negative vibes. But we were about to knock on the client's door – there wasn't time to call them out and start a row. Already both women's level of professionalism was embarrassing and reflected badly not just on me but also on the agency. *Some ladies just do not have a clue how to do this job,* I thought. *They just want to take the money and run.* Clients could sense it and see straight through it.

Then they left the job early without even telling me they were going, leaving me with a group of guys on my own. Luckily the clients were OK – I had been there before and knew them a little. But to walk out on a group booking without telling the one person left that you are leaving is rude, and, more importantly, it's dangerous. When I got back, I told Kim about their early departure. 'That cannot happen again,' I said firmly. 'Do not book me on any more jobs with Kitty and Rachel.' Kim got the message.

The difference between an OK booking and an amazing one is the whole package: looks, skills, personality, energy, humour, affection, connection. To be good at this job is about so much more than taking your clothes off, having sex with a client and then just walking out the door. We work in a feel-good service; I genuinely want my clients to feel better after spending time with me because that in turn makes me feel good. If we, as sex workers, want the respect that we feel we deserve then we also need to show respect back to the client. If a client doesn't respect us then we just don't see that person again and, instead, attract better.

Maybe it's because how successful I am at my job is so dependent on me being able to make instant connections with people, but I really notice how, as a society, we are losing that sense of connection with one another in many different ways. Technology and social media specifically, I'm sure, has played a huge role in this. We are *connected* (through our phones) but not *connecting*. There is a big difference. Maybe this is another reason why internet dating has never been for me. Reducing humans to a series of photos and a few lines of text on a screen and being asked to swipe left or right on them just cannot be good for us. As humans, we are always going to long for some form of connection. Skin-on-skin contact brings humans to life. We crave it.

• • •

Around this time, I had started seeing someone. His name was Jamie. Even though we weren't officially in a relationship, I decided to risk telling him about my job. I just couldn't stand the lie. It did not go down well. We didn't see each other for a while after that.

But, boy, did I pay the price for being honest when we eventually did see each other again! It sounded like he had come to terms with my revelation and we met for drinks in central London. While we were out, a guy who was coming to do some work on the house I was living in had been calling my phone. That's all it took to trigger the argument. Jamie was totally paranoid that it was a client calling me. It really rattled him.

We left the bar and were making our way through Paddington station. He started shouting, 'You're out there getting fucked and sucked!' loud and clear for the whole station to hear. There he was, openly shaming me to the whole world. I wanted the ground to swallow me whole. Before I knew it, a lady with a push bike, dressed head to toe in fluorescents complete with cycle clips and helmet, the whole shebang, bravely tried to intervene. 'You don't have to put up with this!' she kindly and firmly informed me.

'She's brassing herself off!' Jamie shouted back at the cyclist.

I felt like I wanted to die. *Oh God*, I thought to myself, *please no one be filming this. Please no one be uploading this onto social media.* I felt totally vulnerable and as though the whole world was looking on at me in judgement. In that moment, Jamie had won and backed me into submission. I was right back where I'd sworn I'd never be. I felt like the worst person in the world.

Two police officers came marching straight towards us. They separated us for questioning. 'Has there been a history of domestic violence?' the officer asked me. 'No,' I informed him. There hadn't been. He was never abusive, just unstable and paranoid. Luckily, their presence was enough to calm Jamie down. He soon apologised and we were on our way. Needless to say, that 'relationship' didn't go any further.

Thank you to cycle clips lady for trying your best to help. I cannot stand that word 'brass'. It's not as if I ever liked it, but now it makes me shudder. Jamie shouting that word at me aloud in public was a total humiliation.

• • •

This was not my only encounter with the police around this time. I'd been to a party booking with two other ladies at a two-bedroom terraced house on a suburban street. It was the usual situation, to be expected at that time on a Friday evening: a horny group of young guys who had been out all night drinking, snorting cocaine and doing MDMA. After a bit of idle chit chat the lads gravitated towards the lady they were most into and we each found a corner of the house for a moment of intimacy. The guy I was with was tall and toned, smooth chest, great arse (though high as a kite). He watched me touch myself as I lay back and watched him pleasure himself. It was over within minutes. After the hour, the three of us left.

Just as I got in the waiting car to return to the office, a car slowly turned around the corner and began to pull up next to us. I was blinded by their lights. 'What's going on?' I asked my driver.

'Police,' he said.

My heart began to race. 'We'll just be honest with them, yeah?'

'Yeah,' he said as he got out of the car and walked over to them for a chat.

Shit, shit. What if this gets me really in the shit? What if they ask details? How honest should I be?

I tried to look like I was perfectly calm, casually swinging my earphones like I was just doing a normal thing, hanging out in a car on a quiet street in the middle of the night.

The driver returned.

'What did the police say?' I asked.

'He just wanted to know who was in the car.'

The police then drove away and that was the end of it. I began to feel the adrenaline fade. My brush with the law had passed.

To be clear, in case you are not sure, it is not illegal in England, Wales and Scotland to buy or sell sex, though there are laws against soliciting and advertising sexual services, and other things around sex work, like 'brothel keeping' (honestly, the language in these laws is a *delight*). Which means that if you and another sex worker operate from the same flat, even if you are never there at the same time, you could be charged with running a brothel. Some things that could keep sex workers safer are not legal.

The legal framework around selling sex in England, Wales and Scotland means sex work is referred to as being 'partially decriminalised'. If this sounds confusing, it's because it is. But of course it's not just a lack of understanding of the law that keeps some sex workers from reporting crimes against them – or a lack of trust in the police either, although this can certainly be a factor too. It comes back to that stigma. And therefore shame. The thing that kept me sneaking around behind my housemates' back, worried that someone would 'out me', and feeling unable to be honest with so many people in my life. The thing that made me worried about telling the prosecutor in the case of someone who had been violent towards me how we had met.

There was a client I visited in west London many times. One particular summer's day, I had finished the booking, came out of his apartment block and started walking along the pavement when I looked up and saw one of my massage clients. I gulped and tried my best to act natural. I mentally thanked the universe that I was in my casual daytime 'I'm just a regular kind of person' wear. *Big smiles*, I thought. He had already seen me.

'Hi, how are you?' I said as I continued walking past him.

'All right,' was his response, and so we continued.

Out of the corner of my eye, I saw my massage client walk into the same building as my sex work client. 'Shit!' Two worlds colliding.

The next time I saw my massage client at work, I felt the urge to bring up our chance encounter. 'I was out visiting friends who live in the area,' I explained.

'Oh, I just assumed you were at my neighbour's,' he said.

'Oh? What made you think that?' I said curiously.

'He has girls go to his place to massage him.'

Shit, I thought, *why didn't I just say that?* I was just so programmed to hide and deny. There was a reasonable explanation that hadn't even occurred to me. Who knows if the massage client had even thought anything of seeing me in his neighbourhood. I was so conditioned by society's standards, which to me translated as 'Hide who you really are from the rest of the world and live in shame.'

• • •

I was unusually nervous before the first booking with Mark, though I had no idea why.

'But you've done this hundreds of times, you'll be fine!' Kim assured me, bemused at my sudden attack of stage fright.

She was right. It made no sense to feel that nervous.

Soon after, I was standing at the front door of a house on the outskirts of London. When it opened, my jaw dropped to the floor. Mark was one of the most attractive clients that I had ever seen. He was tall and toned, a 'pretty boy' Jude Law type. I tried my best to keep my cool while feeling very glad that my inexplicable nerves had made me pay extra attention to how I looked that day!

Mark soon became a trusted regular and would book me on a weekly basis. I loved being in his company; we had great chemistry. He was a similar to age to me and we shared the same tastes in music. And we both loved to party, of course. The parties were wild; we'd often involve other ladies and party together. Every booking with Mark involved cocaine and alcohol. It was as if we both had our feet firmly on the accelerator.

After spending a wild night in a hotel together – up all night drinking, snorting cocaine, chatting, listening to music, dancing, fucking until the sun rose – Mark had to leave early in the morning for work. I managed to get a late checkout and stayed in bed as long as possible. For this particular booking, because I knew beforehand that I was going to be with the same client all night and by now he was a trusted regular, I had decided to make my own way over and drive. So, when the time came, I checked out of the hotel and made my way over to my car. I went to put the key in the ignition, but something stopped me. I couldn't physically do it. There was no way that I was sober enough drive. My body knew it and my guardian angel knew it.

I got out of the car and informed reception that I'd be taking a cab home and would collect my car in the next few days. I have no idea why I'd thought I'd be OK to drive home. How the hell Mark drove in that state, I'll never know. I've never had an experience like that before or since. I was just not thinking straight that day; the drugs had totally messed with my head. It was another warning sign that the party lifestyle had a shelf life, but not one I was ready to heed yet.

Another booking with Mark in another hotel room. This time, though, something felt really off. It wasn't until we both started to sober up that we realised that the cocaine had been cut with ketamine (horse tranquiliser) and we had both gone into a 'k-hole'.

It was not pleasurable for me at all. Total hell, in fact. When Mark left for work, that hotel room soon began to feel like a prison cell. I had to get out of there and back into my bed as soon as I could. But to do this, I had to get the train across to the other side of London and out again. I must have looked like such a state. It was the journey from hell.

One night, Mark invited me to go to a gig with him. Of course, we took coke. We always did. There we were in the crowd, coked off our faces, and Mark tried to affectionately put his arm around me. In public. It totally threw me. I just did not feel comfortable and paranoia began to set in. That was when it started to dawn on me that perhaps I shouldn't be doing cocaine anymore. It was starting to lose the 'fun' element. The wheels were starting to turn in a new direction as I began questioning myself and my habits. That's the thing with sex work. Drugs are rife within the industry, and I never had to pay a penny for it.

It wasn't just the coke that had made me freak out when Mark touched me in public. I could feel myself starting to fall for him. We had been spending a lot of time together and he even asked if I wanted to go on holiday with him. The boundaries were getting blurred among the chaos of the drugs and alcohol. Developing feelings was certainly starting to feel like a downside to the job. It made things complicated and cost me money. I didn't have high hopes for a future with Mark, but I was only human and could no longer deny that the feelings I was developing for him were very real. I couldn't risk a repeat of Shaun, so I slowly began to distance myself from him. It wasn't until a few months later when he was still messaging me (yes, another faux pas in exchanging numbers with clients while under the influence), asking me to join him with other ladies on party bookings, that I decided to block him. It had all become rather tiresome and I wanted to ensure that I was doing everything I could to protect myself from another 'relationship' disaster.

• • •

My time at Lust was coming to an end. Not all bookings were rainbows and sunshine but on the vast majority, I'd had fun. I was now at the point where I could usually tell when speaking to a prospective client on the phone if we'd click and I had increasingly more confidence in my instincts. Though occasionally I'd slip up. The not-so positive experiences for me usually came in the form of having zero chemistry with the client.

ELIZABETH G.

During one of my weekend shifts, I received a booking that was near to where Shaun lived. I was livid. The thought of going anywhere near there terrified me for obvious reasons. I had already explained this to everyone at Lust and repeatedly told this particular receptionist that I could not do bookings anywhere near where my abusive ex, who I had a restraining order against, lived. But the receptionist didn't seem to care. She was money hungry and willing to risk my safety. I stood up for myself and told her this wasn't OK, that our safety should be the primary concern. This went down like a lead balloon and caused a huge fallout.

It wasn't the first run-in I'd had with her. One morning after I'd been working all through the night and was high as a kite, she had refused to let me back into the office to sleep. By this time, I was temporarily renting a room in the family home of one of my massage clients. There was no way I could return at 7 a.m. wide-eyed and still buzzing from the night before. The other receptionists understood and would let me back in the office to sleep it off during the day. But this receptionist refused. My driver couldn't wait with me until she left so I was forced to hang out at the local service station on my own. In an industry that encourages drug and alcohol use, this treatment was shocking. I take full responsibility for my actions – I am certainly not blaming anyone else for my choice to drink and take cocaine – and yet the fact remains that a lot of the work was 'party bookings'. If I were to say that I didn't drink or do drugs, it was frowned upon, like I was being difficult. In my view, therefore, the agency had a duty of care.

This incident prompted me to move on from Lust. I was grateful for the years there, but I am a firm believer that everything happens for a reason. Sometimes these challenging situations force us to move in a new direction. I had become comfortable at Lust and staying in your comfort zone is a dangerous place to be. There is no chance for growth or opportunity there. I was forced to move on because I stood up for what I believed in. I stood up for my own safety. In doing this, I was putting a very strong message out there to the universe about my worth. And, in return, the universe led me to a high-end agency in Mayfair.

CHAPTER EIGHT

HIGH-END

I was back at the farm having dinner with my family. It was a lovely night and we were all getting on well. I felt happy and at peace, even though there was a lot riding on what I had planned for the next day. Which was not something I could have shared with my family, of course. So I smiled and enjoyed their company and tried to be in the moment.

My finances were running dangerously low. I needed a new job and I had set my sights on Archie's, a high-end agency in Mayfair. It would be a big step up from Lust and a lot more money. For this, I needed some flawless professional photos. So I had used the remaining money I had to set up a photoshoot, to get some great shots that I could send to Archie's and some of the other high-end agencies.

I barely had enough money for petrol to get back to London, let alone for any slip-ups along the way. So the next morning, I was up at 6 a.m. and in the car and on the road to London at 7.30 a.m. It was a perfect journey; the sun was shining, the roads were clear. Even driving through rush hour wasn't too painful. Anything could have gone wrong during that journey; my car could have broken down (it had issues and had let me down before), tube lines could have been down (they too hadn't exactly been reliable lately), I could have overslept and not heard my alarm. I was prepared for anything and everything, while trying to keep my cool and not let anxiety take over. But it all ran smoothly. It was meant to be.

I arrived in central London early in the end. The studio was beautiful and the make-up artist very professional. Everything just fitted perfectly that day. The photographer even sat with me after the photoshoot, chose the photos and edited them with me (something that usually took him a week).

ELIZABETH G.

He then gave me three extra photos for free. Sure, he was a little too flirty and tried his best to barter for a free kinky massage, but I brushed this aside and was still grateful for his help.

So that was it; the photos were edited and ready to be sent out. I was very happy with them. I felt like my luck was finally changing, like this was a defining moment for me. I felt blessed. After starving myself all day, I went straight to McDonald's to stuff my face.

Shortly after, a friend that I had worked with at Lust called. 'What are you doing now? I have a job for you if you are interested. It's only in Tower Bridge. It's just to sit and chat with him for a couple of hours while I go on another job. Casual clothes are fine. He'll pay £400.'

I couldn't believe it! And so off I went. My luck was finally up again. I went from being down to my last £10 to having £400 in my bank account. How life can be full of pleasant surprises when you don't give up.

The next day I received the text to say that Archie's were happy to take me on, starting the following week. I cried tears of relief. It had been a tough few months but now I felt like my perseverance and resilience were starting to pay off. I remained a little cautious, worried that it could all fall through, but it was at least something positive to focus on for the week ahead. Maybe it was just luck, maybe it was my new-found belief in the law of attraction. Whatever it was, it was working. I believed in myself. In my self-worth. In my own staying power and in my persistence. I was taking action and I was daring myself to dream.

• • •

My first day working at Archie's had me beaming with excitement. I decided to work under the name Olivia. By this time, I had a few years of experience working as a sex worker behind me. I knew the drill, understood the assignment. This agency was slightly different in that I would be working from a hotel room rather than have a driver take me around the outskirts of London to clients' homes and hotels. I much preferred the idea of having my own space in a hotel room, plus the pay was better and I got a bigger piece of the pie – the agency took 30 per cent of what we made. Most bookings would be incalls but I was also to expect some outcalls. I had only ever done outcalls before so, with less travelling to do, I was looking forward to having a bit more of a balance and more time to myself. I'd been working less and less at my massage job and decided to take a break when I started at Archie's.

The best part of all was that I got to choose my own hours! I remain convinced that working hours to suit my own schedule is the secret to happiness. At Lust, there had been two choices – day shift or night shift. But Archie's offered a flexibility that I could only ever have dreamt of. There was no limit or minimum or set times. I chose when I worked. No more graveyard shifts working all through the night and sleeping throughout the day. I was so grateful for my new-found freedom.

In the beginning, most days I worked 2 p.m. to midnight, Monday to Thursday, depending on what I had going on from one week to the next. Rather than get another house share in London, I decided to spend the money on hotel stays instead. After spending a few days in London working, I'd pack up my stuff, check out of the hotel and drive back to Bedfordshire to stay on the farm with my brother for a few days of R&R. By this time, my father had retired so he and my mother moved to a house in the neighbouring village. This yo-yoing back and forth, living out of a suitcase, continued for about eighteen months.

I immediately noticed a difference in the clients now that I was at a high-end agency. As you would maybe expect, they appeared to be much more professional: doctors, lawyers, property tycoons, financiers, entrepreneurs, creatives, usually in their forties and fifties, which I preferred. The younger clients in their twenties were never my favourite bookings. They often had a different attitude towards women. Some didn't know how to respect a woman and their knowledge of a woman's body was limited, simply due to lack of experience. No matter how good-looking they were, it didn't make much difference to me. It was experience that turned me on.

My first day at Archie's was one of the busiest days I've ever had, with back-to-back clients all day. I went from zero to ding ding ding very quickly. The last booking of the day was an outcall to a client's home in Knightsbridge. I felt totally overwhelmed as I entered the immaculate building and walked up the spiral staircase to the first-floor apartment. I was engulfed in marble – marble everywhere! Marble flooring, marble walls, marble statues. It reminded me of the fancy London hotels from my days working for Erotica Massage, except this was a private building, where people lived.

I knocked on the door. As the client opened it something felt a little 'off' from the get-go. I didn't get a sense of the warm, buzzing energy that I had felt from clients all day. Still, I proceeded into the property. The client handed me the cash, which I counted, of course. Then, when I was satisfied with the payment, I notified reception that the booking had started. As we were sitting side by side on a pair of thrones, the client turned to me and said very bluntly: 'I'm sorry, but you look nothing like your pictures.' I was totally shocked. In all the years that I had been doing this, I had never had this reaction. I loved my new photos and all my clients so far had seemed very happy to meet me.

'So you want me to leave?' I said nervously, trying not to show my panic.

'Yes,' he said.

I called reception and explained the situation. They were very understanding, thankfully. It was agreed that the client would pay a cancellation fee and I would give some of the money back.

As soon as I could, I bolted out of the door and into a cab back to the hotel. This was not an ideal way to end my first day. During the cab journey, I called reception again, who were so wonderfully supportive and understanding: 'He's just being a dick, don't worry about it.' That was exactly what I needed to hear after feeling so mortified by the client. I'd wanted to make a good impression, so to have this experience at the end of what had previously been a very positive day felt like a defeat. Fast forward to seven years later and I have not had an incident like that since. That experience taught me that the most exciting and extravagant venues are not always the best bookings. Sometimes clients with silly amounts of money are the worst. Not always, but sometimes. It was a very tough lesson learnt that day. The positive was that my intuition telling me that there was something about this particular client that was not good had been right. On reflection, I was glad that he asked me to leave. My intuition, my sense of people, is one of the most powerful tools I have. I felt like I had dodged a bullet that day.

•••

It didn't take long for me to build up a trusted list of regular clients. I was growing in confidence and really starting to find my feet while working at Archie's. My bookings began to soar. The balance of incalls and outcalls was perfect and I was starting to fall head over heels in love with London. It reminded me a little of that feeling I'd had when I'd first moved to Hampstead before my relationship with Shaun had sabotaged it all.

I loved the adventures of going to outcall bookings at high-end hotels. I learnt the art of boldly walking into a hotel lobby while smiling sweetly at the reception staff. My killer smile and innocent looks made it much easier to convince them that I was a regular visitor. Discretion and professionalism are a key part of my job, especially with outcall bookings. I also learnt to always insist that Archie's receptionists checked before my arrival if a key card was needed for the lift. I never wanted to put myself in that awkward situation of pressing the button and the lift going nowhere. I didn't want to make myself stand out from the crowd.

I got to meet people from all walks of life with interesting stories to tell. It wasn't a case of just having sex and getting out of there. Talking to the clients was an important part of the job and I realised that they were often people I could learn from. I loved the excitement of it all: the build-up, the meeting for the first time and exploring each other as two strangers. There were lots of dinner dates too. At the end of the encounter, I would leave a very happy customer and with a wad of cash in my handbag, taking an evening cab ride back to the hotel among the bright lights of London, feeling the energy of life all around me. In the morning before my shift, I often took a walk around Hyde Park. Though I was still commuting to and from Bedfordshire, London was beginning to feel like home.

In the early days of Archie's, I began doing incalls from a hotel notorious for sex workers. 'Let's just say it's for ladies of the night,' said a taxi driver. I acted innocent – despite having just been picked up from the front entrance. 'Oh gosh, really?'

Playing the dumb blonde was still my thing. I had learnt to use it to my advantage. People would underestimate me and I would take great pleasure in either proving them wrong or getting away with whatever I wanted. I didn't work from the notorious hotel for long as I soon cottoned on that some clients deliberately avoided going there due to the hotel's notoriety. The *Daily Mail* once described it as 'ten floors of whores' and published pictures of sex workers' profiles, their faces not even blurred out. Outing sex workers like that should be illegal. Publishing those types of articles only makes sex workers more vulnerable and open to abuse.

• • •

That summer of 2018 felt like the summer of love. William and Kate had their third child, Prince Louis; Prince Harry married Meghan Markle; England got through to the semi-finals of the FIFA World Cup and women in Saudi Arabia were given the right to drive. My close childhood friend, Lara, got married in the most idyllic 'midsummer's dream' ceremony and I enjoyed reunions by the coast with other very special childhood friends.

My business is a fickle one. It's unpredictable and the volume of bookings ebbs and flows, often without there being an obvious reason. However, there are a few factors that do have a noticeable impact. For example, when the World Cup was on that summer, bookings would go dead while England were playing (I was pleased; I wanted to watch the match). Afterwards, bookings would begin to soar regardless of whether England won or lost. Ramadan always had an obvious effect on earnings. (Business also often booms just before school holidays and drops off during them, for example – make of that what you will.) I would soon learn that summertime in central London was, generally, a very lucrative period. The economy was good. Despite the ongoing Brexit negotiations, London was thriving.

My first booking in the Savoy left a lasting impression. We pulled up to the entrance of the iconic London hotel and I hopped out of the cab to be greeted by a very friendly and smartly dressed doorman: top hat and tails, the usual for a high-end London hotel.

As I entered the foyer, memories of my booking at the Dorchester for Erotica Massage came flooding back to me. So much had changed since then. I was older and more experienced. I had grown in confidence. I boldly made my way over to the lift and up to the client's room. When I reached his floor, I swiftly changed from my flats into heels (a new trick – it made getting around London so much more comfortable). I was greeted by a larger-than-life character who had booked the most impressive suite I had ever seen. The client was from LA and worked in film. It was one of my first bookings with an American.

I have come to learn that American clients are the dream. They're among the most easy-going, easily pleased clients I have ever had the pleasure of meeting. Perhaps it's because sex work is so highly illegal over in the States (with some exceptions), so for many coming to the UK, they are just happy that they can book a sex worker without having to worry about being arrested.

In the cab on the way back to my hotel, the driver said to me, 'You look happy. I can see it in your eyes and your smile. I used to be a hairdresser for many years and I can always tell how someone's feeling or to stay away from them, you know?'

'Yeah, I'm a massage therapist, it's a similar thing, tuning in with people's energy,' I said. Which was true in sentiment, if inaccurate in terms of facts.

Truth is, I was happy. Incredibly happy. I was earning good money and doing a job that I loved. It was a beautiful sunny day in London and I was grateful to simply have air in my lungs and a beating heart. In that moment it felt good to be alive.

From the Mandarin Oriental in Knightsbridge to the ME hotel in the Strand, I was soon racking up a list of high-end hotel experiences. Visiting the finest hotels and restaurants in and around Mayfair was always fun.

A visit to the Connaught had me totally mesmerised. I'd never heard of this hotel before the booking. To a woman from the countryside, it seemed to be a bit more off the beaten track compared to the likes of the Dorchester, the Ritz and the Savoy. The client had booked one of the apartments. Not your regular apartment: three storeys, grand piano, fluffy slippers and feet cushions on either side of the bed. Immaculate attention to detail. It was one of the most beautiful apartments I had ever seen.

However, the bookings in the most luxurious surroundings were not always the ones that particularly stuck in my mind. It was all very nice, of course, but what really mattered, when it came down to 'business', was how the client was. Clean, well-groomed, polite, respectful clients were always favourable. Skills and chemistry on top of that were an added bonus. The best bookings have been with the most giving clients, clients who I naturally click with, and who want to have a bit of a chat first. Some clients bring me flowers, jewellery, chocolates, fruit (I'm very happy to receive any food in general!). Other clients have been very talented at giving oral, and very eager to do so. I love the clients who want to massage me as well as me massage them; the clients who want to go out for dinner first and catch up. Essentially, those who see me as a human being, not some toy to treat as they please just because they are paying.

I have had clients say to me, 'Well, I'm the one paying', while pointing to themselves, indicating that they can do whatever they want. Sorry, darlings, it doesn't work like that. Would you treat your lawyer exactly how you wish just because you are paying them? No. The same goes for sex workers. It is a service. It is a profession. You treat us with respect no matter how much you are paying. That is non-negotiable.

I was starting to meet more and more clients that I clicked well with and would see on a regular basis. When I felt like I 'knew' a client, I would often be comfortable exploring with them – bondage, submission and roleplay. My master's in acting had not gone to waste! And of course, there were still lots of party bookings, with free-flowing alcohol, cocaine and my all-time favourite, Mandy (MDMA). It was at Archie's where I gained most of my experiences in duo bookings with fellow sex workers. Party bookings with colleagues were always a fun night.

And yes, there have been many random requests over the years. Time spent with a sex worker is, after all, time spent in a safe space for clients to explore their inner-most desires without judgement (all within agreed, respected boundaries, of course). It must have been just after Brexit when a client requested that I wear a T-shirt saying 'Keep calm and vote Conservative' while fucking him from behind with a strap-on. I got a lot of enjoyment from wearing a strap-on. There was a certain empowerment that came with it. In the early days of being a sex worker, I was very much a submissive type. However, in more recent years I am certainly happier being in charge and laying down the law.

While working at the 'hotel of notoriety' I met Charlie. He came across as 'one of the lads' but was well groomed, polite and friendly with great energy. He was also incredibly handsome and very muscular with great shoulders and arms – as always a turn-on for me. It's usually the thing I notice before anything else. I can pick a good set of shoulders out of a crowd almost instantly.

I first met Charlie while I was on a detox. The party bookings had been going a bit crazy and I could feel my body urging me to take a break. I think Charlie was a bit surprised that I didn't want to drink or take drugs with him but he accepted it. Years later, he told me that he thought I was some kind of extreme vegan when we first met, all because I was on a detox. How wrong he was!

We clicked instantly and ended up in the casino that night. And thus began many years of great sex, parties, trips to the pub, dinner dates, dancing, adventures, advice on life and discussing intently the affairs of the day. Charlie soon became one of my most loyal regulars. Through my ups and downs, he has been there. Rightly or wrongly, in more recent years I see him less as a client and more as a very good friend with very good benefits. While experience has taught me that romantic relationships between sex workers and clients rarely ever work out, in special circumstances, friendship can. Charlie is the dream.

A lot of clients will happily sit and chat and talk about anything from politics and current affairs to the latest scandal and I happily oblige. Again, probably surprising to anyone who thinks sex work is literally just about having sex. I've had a lot of interesting, intellectual conversations over the years and I've learnt a lot from my clients, about business, about finances, about investing. Intelligence turns me on.

ELIZABETH G.

The only danger with developing a good relationship with a regular client is that some can became obsessive. When this has happened I have found it uncomfortable, never flattering. It reminded me of Shaun, even if the client was otherwise nothing like him. It was during this summer of love in 2018 that I met Fabio. He was a kind soul; I could see that as soon as we met. He would book me on a regular basis; we'd sit and chat over a cup of tea. He liked to be sensual, which was always music to my ears. But over time, I could feel him latching on to me, like a noose around my neck getting tighter and tighter. 'We are connected,' he'd say insistently and repeatedly. It started to scare me.

I called Archie to make him aware of the situation. I had worked for the agency for a few months by the time I met Archie in person. He was a very likeable character. An old-school gentleman type, he was always smartly dressed and well groomed, as well as professional and buzzing with positive vibes. Archie was always so great to talk to, so understanding. 'Darling, you've got to enjoy yourself. If you don't think that you and the client are going to click at the beginning of the booking, then simply give the money back and ask them to leave,' he'd tell me. After I explained about the situation with Fabio, that I had a bad feeling about it, he ended up going on my banned list. Reception were made aware and I never saw him again. Once I made that decision, I felt as though a huge weight had been lifted.

I continued to build more regular clients, learning more and more, having lots of adventures with a few faux pas along the way. I had migrated from working from the hotel of notoriety to serviced studio apartments recommended by the agency. Basement studios became my preference as they usually came with their own entrance separate to the rest of the building. This meant that clients didn't have to worry about getting past a reception desk and I didn't have to worry about the risk of being quizzed by hotel staff. One day, however, I got the shock of my life when, while I was in the middle of going down on a client, the cleaner opened the door. No warning sign, no knocking, no nothing. Just waltzed in like she was entering her own home! Out of the corner of my eye, I saw her enter the apartment, heading towards the bedroom. With the client naked and spreadeagled on the bed, I jumped up. 'What the hell?!' I barked at her. As soon as she realised, she was out the door, never to return.

I freaked out and rang Archie. I was panicking that somehow, just because of one cleaner, my secret would be out to the whole world. Or at the very least she'd tell the hotel and they'd ask me to leave. I never, ever wanted to be kicked out of a hotel – I'd heard the rumours of it happening and never wanted it to be me. Once I'd calmed down I realised that, to the cleaner, for all she knew, we were just a couple having sex. She didn't see any transaction. She just saw a regular sex act. But again, the fear, the shame, had blurred my vision. I had conditioned myself to the point where I believed that I was doing something so wrong that any outsider looking in would know immediately what was going on and hang me out to dry. Of course, nothing happened, and I was not asked to leave.

...

I've had the pleasure of sampling tastes from many different countries. But there really is just something about the French. That familiar stereotype of the French being quite the connoisseurs when it comes to sex is for good reason! I've never had a bad experience with a French man. 'So, you've never had a French loveeeur?' one asked me as he pounded me left, right and centre, in every position possible, his body toned, taut and all muscle – absolute fireworks! By the time the booking ended, I looked like I had been dragged through a bush ten times over. Always a sign of a good session! Rosy-pink cheeks, glowing from ear to ear, mascara halfway down my face and my long blonde locks looking like a backcomb from the 1980s gone horribly wrong. It's fair to say, that was a good day in the 'office'!

As sensual as I am, on some days, with the right client, I just wanted to be bent over, dominated and have someone fuck the crap out of me. Not in an aggressive manner; still connected, of course, and communicating through our bodies, through our movements. But some days I would wake up and something very animalistic would come over me. I would be like, 'Take me, I'm yours.' That's where Mr Dom came in. Incredible. Insatiable. Every time. He seemed to bring out a certain side of me that I didn't know I had. We'd both switch between being submissive and dominant. That's the great thing about sex work – with trusted regulars, it has allowed me to really explore myself sexually. With some clients, we'd learn and grow together – through foreplay, roleplay, submission, dominance. I learnt from them and they learnt from me.

One rainy afternoon (the rain makes me very horny; something about it feels very primal – sex in the rain in my wellies, now that's my ideal!), I was delighted to see a booking from Mr Dom pop up. It was always a pleasure to see him as I knew I was guaranteed to have a good time. While Mr Dom took a shower, I laid a selection of restraints on the bed for him to choose from. I removed my secretary wear to reveal my red lace lingerie, stockings and suspenders and waited patiently. He walked out of the shower, his body wet and glistening, and strode straight over to me. No hesitation. Proudly displaying his rock-hard cock. He pulled me into him and grabbed my behind. Our tongues began to intertwine. I slowly began to stroke the back of his neck with my fingernails, waking up his erogenous zones. He removed my bra and released my breasts.

He didn't hesitate to caress my nipples with his tongue as I began to lightly stroke his cock. That excited me and I had to restrain myself from pushing him onto the bed and straddling him in that very moment. I crouched down to his groin and slowly started licking his balls and teasing his cock, looking up at him with a naughty glint in my eye. I had him right where I wanted him. I saw him peering into the mirror behind me, which gave him a fine view of my behind. As I went deeper with his cock in my mouth, he tilted his head back and I could feel his sense of relief. He had been waiting some time for that moment. That first moment when I slowly began to put my mouth around his cock, using my tongue to stimulate the tip.

He ordered me to stand against the door and raise my arms above my head. My nipples began to harden with the excitement and anticipation of what he'd do next. He strapped my wrists into the overhead restraints and blindfolded me. He then brought out my spreader bar, forcing my legs to open wider. He strapped in my ankles and I accept that, in that moment, he was in charge and I was his submissive. I felt the warmth of his breath all over my body as he began to tease every part of me. I was getting wetter and wetter as his tongue began to stimulate my clitoris. I was squirming with excitement and feeling more and more ravenous for him.

He whispered in my ear, 'How much do you want my cock?'

'I want your cock throbbing inside me from behind. I've missed your cock!' I said.

After teasing me to the point where I was quivering all over, he removed the restraints and I guided him over to the wall. With my back to him, showing him my arse, which he loved so much, I said softly, 'I need your cock inside me now,' looking over my shoulder.

Following my orders, he rubbered up and then slipped his hard, throbbing cock inside me; I was now dripping in anticipation. He took me from behind. My body tingled all over as his cock slid in. I flicked my head back with relief as though I had been waiting for that moment for some time too.

We gained momentum, as I felt myself get wetter and wetter until he could hear me squelch. He pounded me harder and harder from behind, whispering in my ear while he had me pinned against the wall, my arms in the air.

'Harder!' I insisted. He went in deeper, harder and faster. I felt his tongue on my neck as he pulsated harder and faster, and I began to cum – 'I'm cumming!' He pulled me in harder. A moment of relief.

We moved to the bed and I lay on my back, legs in the air so he could go even deeper inside of me. 'Pin me down and fuck me!' He willingly followed orders. Holding me down and going deeper still. Our bodies were glistening, sweat pouring, the headboard banging louder against the window. He groaned and, with one last thrust, I felt his cock inside me begin to pulsate as he blew his load. We collapsed on the bed, rosy cheeked and with our heads in the clouds. I looked up to the sky and thanked the universe for the life that I was living.

• • •

A typical day at work starts with checking that I am fully stocked: condoms, check. Lube, check. Baby wipes, check. BV gel, cranberry tablets (I have no time for cystitis), fresh towels, men's shower gel, men's body spray, mouthwash. I'd make sure the flat I was using was clean and tidy, smelling fresh, sometimes lighting candles. I'd get out my lingerie and heels, roleplay outfits and toys. Then press play on my specially created sexy playlist. Once a client arrives and the payment has been made, I show them to the shower. This is non-negotiable. On the rare instances a client has had an issue with getting in the shower, it's always been a red flag for how the booking would go. Poor hygiene to a sex worker is a mark of disrespect. As Archie would say: 'Please never feel obliged to proceed with a booking if the client is smelly or rude or dirty, or indeed makes you feel uncomfortable in ANY way. There are enough fun, clean and respectful clients out there for you to share your time with. Dirty, rude clients can book elsewhere. We only want clean, respectful clients booking with our agency.'

Music has always been the key for me and helps me get into the zone. Aside from the hair, make-up, stockings and suspender sets, music is a powerful way of bringing out the character of Olivia. It's all part of my preparation and mentally honing in on that part of myself. Like an actor preparing for a role. Especially on days when I was feeling nervous, I'd crank up the music, have a dance, bounce, sway, gyrate around my flat in my heels and lingerie. The playlist has been tweaked and changed over the years but there are some songs that have remained trusted favourites: 'Black Velvet' by Alannah Myles, 'Breathe on Me' by Britney Spears, 'Glory Box' by Portishead, 'Erotica' by Madonna and 'Partition' by Beyoncé. Anything with a deep bass line sung by a woman.

'The thing that makes you so addictive is that you genuinely seem to enjoy what you do.' Years after our first meeting, one of my trusted regulars gave me just the ego boost that I needed to hear. He was right. I genuinely loved my job – depending on the client; some days I was in acting mode more than others. But with him, it was genuine. Absolute fireworks. Antonio just knew how to make me weak at the knees. And he did have me at my knees for him for many years. I'd always thought something was wrong with me because I couldn't squirt. That was until I met Antonio.

He'd have me squirming with pleasure, drenching the sheets every time. Some days, there'd be a puddle on the floor. So now when a client asks me, 'Can you squirt?' I bat it straight back to them. 'The question is, can you *make* me squirt?' And they never can. Antonio just knew which buttons to push. His accuracy and precision were on point every single time. His skills were unbeatable. We progressed over the years, exploring each other's bodies. He was always in charge. I was happy to oblige and be his submissive. He was my master and I was his subject. To date, he is the most sensual dominating man I have ever met. The chemistry between us was insatiable and I thanked my lucky stars every time I had the pleasure of meeting him.

I was surprised at how busy bookings were during the day – lots of lunchtime quickies. So, I began to adjust my hours accordingly, starting earlier and finishing earlier. I slowly started to wean myself off the super-late-night bookings and began starting around 11 a.m. and finishing around 9 p.m. It made a huge difference to my mindset. I was beginning to feel less burnt out. Plus, the more sensual and more confident I was becoming, the more sensual clients I was attracting. I was slowly beginning to learn the art of tease, the art of tantric sex. Of building up to the point where I had the client squirming, begging me to make him cum.

The door to my sensual side really opened up when I met Hunter. He was a tipper and a gift bearer, which always made me feel super special. He was tall and smoulderingly handsome. The stereotypical tall, dark, handsome man, actually. Always suited and booted, always smartly dressed. As soon as he walked through the door, he was right there with me. Eyes on me. Connected. As with Antonio, he'd book me for a few hours at a time. We'd start by chatting and having a catch-up, sometimes with tea and cake, sometimes with a glass of wine, discussing current affairs and what was going on in the world at the time. We'd build things up slowly, taking our time. He'd always bring massage oils with him and would insist on beginning by giving me a very slow and sensual massage. Heaven. There was something about taking things very slowly, about being very giving on both sides, that really turned me on. To build and build and build while exploring each other's bodies had me quivering all over.

• • •

I was finally earning good money and the days when I was constantly worried about how to pay my bills seemed long past. I could afford an M&S food shop whenever I wanted – the true mark of success to me! The vast majority of clients paid in cash. Only with my trusted regulars did I let them do a bank transfer. During one of my weekly trips to the bank to pay in my earnings, a mega bitch sitting behind the counter began quizzing me. It completely threw me. I saw her clock my manicured nails, the thousands of pounds I was paying in, and I felt like she had it in for me straight away.

'Where's the money come from?' she said bluntly while looking me up and down, clearly thinking she was being subtle.

'Work. I'm a massage therapist,' I said.

She grilled me further and began asking more about my massage work. I understand that this may be a standard thing for some banks and they have to be vigilant about money laundering and things like that, but it was her whole attitude; her aura and look of judgement stank. By the end of it, she had me backed into a corner, giving her my phone number to book a massage. Of course, she never messaged me. She never had any intention of messaging or calling me, she just wanted to bring me down. Well, that day it worked. When I left the bank, I burst into tears.

If I worked in a more 'acceptable' profession, I would have gone straight to her manager and lodged a complaint. But because I was a sex worker, I felt like I couldn't in case it brought about more questions. Her judgement made me feel awful. After that incident, I started paying into the machine. I don't why I didn't think of it at the time, but I should have just given her my accountant's details and asked her to quiz him instead.

I was really fortunate in that I had found a wonderful accountant. They are crucial for many people who are self-employed but hard to find in my profession. Not everyone is going to be comfortable with knowing all about the sorts of essential items we claim on expenses! It took a few bad eggs to find him but eventually I got there and I have stuck with him ever since. He knows all about my profession and has never once judged me or shown any kind of bias. He's always professional, always reassuring, and gives great advice.

• • •

Overnight bookings were beginning to roll in. Meeting clients for drinks in the hotel bar was always a nice way to kick-start the evening, although experience had taught me to be cautious about meeting clients in public spaces, especially in the evening when I'd be dressed up and in heels. I'd always give a description of what I was wearing beforehand and would get a description back, so I didn't end up going up to a random stranger. But there was always an element of feeling like you were walking straight into the unknown. Over time, I have learnt to have confidence with it. 'Hi! So nice to see you! How have you been?' pecking them on both cheeks as if we had been friends for years. Blending in among the tourists. Always professional, always discreet.

However, I once met a client in a Kensington hotel who was clearly quite a bit older than me. We got into the lift and another couple got in at the last minute. The client proceeded to ask me,

'So, where are you from?'

I could have died. 'London,' I just said softly, hoping that the ground would swallow me up whole, while giving the client a 'don't you dare ask me any more questions while we are in this lift!' look. I thought it must have been so obvious what was going on.

Another time, I was out at the pub with Mark, the regular I had become too close to when I was at Lust (and as a result had to stop doing bookings with him). We got chatting to a couple of people and one of them asked, 'So how did you guys meet?'

I was not prepared for that and it completely threw me, sending me into an internal panic. 'We work together,' Mark said. But by then, I had gone bright red and our new-found friends at the pub could see that something didn't quite add up.

Another evening, I went to meet a client for a dinner date. He was from Switzerland and visiting the UK for a work conference. We met in Chelsea. The conversation didn't exactly flow at dinner and, as much as I tried, there were a lot of awkward silences. As the cab pulled up to the hotel, the client got out first, with me closely following behind. As soon as we stepped out, the client saw his colleagues standing right outside. He didn't say anything but I picked up on a vibe straight away and made a swift manoeuvre to the other side of the entrance and pretended to be on my phone. The client had a brief chat with them and walked straight into the hotel. I waited a few minutes. I was trying to decide what to do when one of his colleagues came over and started talking to me. 'So you are here for the conference too?' she said, smiling at me.

'No,' I said, smiling back. My mind emptied and in that moment I couldn't think of anything else to say.

After waiting a little longer, I decided to walk in and head up to the client's room. As I entered the bustling reception area, I saw the client talking to another group of colleagues. I walked straight past him as though we were strangers and got into the lift. The client met me outside his door soon after. 'You did good,' he assured me.

Occasionally, a booking would bring me crashing back down to earth. It wasn't often but, as with any job, I'd have my good days and occasional bad days. This particular client was called Simon and he was looking for a submissive–dominant experience. He was dominant, I was to be his submissive. He explained that he wanted to dominate me and tie me up. He had brought red lipstick with him so that he could write on me and candles so that he could pour hot candle wax on me. There is no way that I would proceed with this type of booking today. I make it crystal clear to clients that I am very much into a sensual girlfriend experience, not into anything aggressive or degrading. But back then, I didn't know about boundaries; I was never taught about implementing healthy boundaries in any relationship, let alone with a client. I thought my role was to please and I didn't prioritise myself.

The client proceeded to tie me up, pulling the rope tighter and tighter until I realised that there was no way I'd be able to get out. I asked him to untie me, which he did. He then wrote all over my face and body with the red lipstick. The candle wax I didn't mind; I actually quite liked the feeling. After he left, I looked at myself in the mirror: 'slut' and 'whore' had been written all over me. Simon was not the client for me and he went straight onto my banned list.

Shortly after, I asked one of my regular clients, who was a therapist, why a man would want to do that. The first thing he said straight away without hesitation was 'mother issues'. He continued, 'Or, at the very least, issues with women. Perhaps he was rejected by women in his younger years.'

That type of booking was not representative of who I was as a sex worker. I was still learning. Always learning. But back then my boundaries were blurred among the drugs, alcohol and hangovers.

•••

I had been staying at a colleague's flat for a couple of weeks while she was away on holiday. I absolutely loved it. I had my own space in London and could work from home. I was growing increasingly tired of all the toing and froing between London and the farm. It had been around eighteen months now – I was constantly on the road and living out of a suitcase. I was literally travelling between two worlds: between my childhood home and country life and sex work and city life. I was living a classic double life. Some days, I'd wake up having panic attacks. Having secrets is corrosive. It does something very unhealthy to our inner psyche.

The feeling of having to hide my life and live in secret did not sit well with me. In all other areas of my life, I have always been pretty open and honest. It gives me a sense of freedom to get things out and be direct with people, rather than pussyfooting around things. But hiding this secret was now really getting to me. The travel wasn't helping. I longed for a weekend where I could just be still or go for a walk in the park and ground myself, not be driving up and down the M1. I began to envision myself settling in west London. London was really beginning to feel like home.

Bookings were plentiful and I was starting to build up my savings. I felt like I was on a good path. Increasingly I was seeing my profession as a lucrative business with huge opportunities and myself as a businesswoman. I started to set my sights higher. Something in me was changing, emerging. I still didn't have it all figured out, but I was beginning to set my sights on new ventures. I was feeling more grounded and began to have a very clear vision of the direction I wanted my life to go in. I wanted to start investing in property.

I was also realising that the partying was getting a bit too much. I wanted to tone it down. I began to cleanse out 'friends' that I partied with. Looking back, it was the only way and one of the wisest decisions I have ever made. I was learning to step away from the crowd and move in a different direction. I wasn't afraid to be different. I wasn't afraid to hustle. Plus, the scars from Shaun were still well and truly there – I still wanted to make sure that I did everything I could to ensure that I'd never have to rely on a partner for finances ever again. I had to be brave and start moving against the grain. That took a lot of courage. That was when things really began to change.

CHAPTER NINE
MOMENTUM

I moved to west London permanently just after the summer of 2019. I had been working with Archie's for over two years and was looking forward to settling in a part of the city that I had fallen madly in love with. I was thirty-six years old and ready to once again say goodbye to the farm and settle into a place of my own. A place that no one could take away from me or kick me out of. Where I could be free to express my true self, cook whatever food I fancied, play my music as loud as I wanted, dance and sing to my heart's content. Thus began a love affair with west London. The people, the food, the eccentrics, the history, the architecture, the whole ambience. I loved the old romance vibe that came with west London. Almost like stepping back in time.

I'm an old soul at heart. I loved learning about the history, admiring architecture and imagining how life was all those years ago. How life was for women like me. I began retracing the footsteps of sex workers throughout history. I know that I was romanticising to an extent – life was horrible and precarious for many sex workers who had no protection and no recourse to the law. But for some women in history, sex work allowed them to transcend humble beginnings and amass wealth and power. For example, Catherine Walters, aka 'Skittles'. In the late Victorian era, she was a well-known courtesan who set fashion trends.[6] Her perfect figure and riding skills would draw huge crowds on Rotten Row in Hyde Park. Aristocratic ladies began copying her style and it was there in Hyde Park where she began making connections to various clientele and working her way up through society. Her clients included intellectuals, politicians, aristocrats and even, it's thought, the Prince of Wales, who became King Edward VII. She was very discreet and loyal to her clients – she never confirmed or denied rumours. She retired a wealthy woman of society in 1890. Not bad for a woman from a lower-middle class background born many miles from the capital in Liverpool.

Only a few months ago, I visited her home in Mayfair. It was such a surreal feeling as I stood outside reading her blue plaque and imagining the experiences and parties that went on there. The people, the music, the fashion, the language, the sexual debauchery. It made me feel at home and reassured to know that there were so many other women out there throughout history like me. Even if I couldn't help but think about how little progress we had made since then. In fact, had we gone backwards? I couldn't imagine people these days looking up to a sex worker in the way that Catherine Walters was admired.

The road I lived on was lined with beautiful Victorian terraces – crisp, white buildings fronted with large pillars that towered over either side of the front doors. They'd once been home to the upper-middle class before being divided up into individual apartments. London is so rich in history; echoes of the past are everywhere, on every street, on every corner. After living in Australia, I had learnt not to take British heritage for granted. I loved the history of London and I loved learning. I became a history nerd.

The part of west London where I settled was home to people from all cultures and ethnicities, vibrant with life. I fed off the energy of being surrounded by people day and night. In the height of summer, the buzz of life would continue well past midnight.

I always felt safe there. Much safer than living out in the sticks. I liked the reassurance of life around me at all hours. Eyes everywhere. Witnesses. Now, when I go home to the countryside or for a break away, I struggle to sleep with silence around me. I find the silence deafening. It has me on edge.

It was a transient area, with people constantly passing through. This meant that I could blend in very easily and my movements went unnoticed. My neighbours didn't give a shit about me and I didn't give a shit about them. It was quite the contrast, returning from my small hometown, with nosey middle-aged locals quizzing me on my every move, to my flat in London, crossing paths with one of my neighbours on the stairs and smiling at him, only to be greeted with a grunt. No smile, no 'how are you?' *I bloody love London. It's so good to be back!* I thought.

I moved into a mezzanine flat – high ceilings, floor-to-ceiling windows, a large balcony, four-poster bed, mirror. It all felt very Parisian. It was the kind of flat that I *wanted* to have sex in. A place where I could really let myself loose and immerse myself in my work. A place to hone my craft and develop my skills. I knew a lot of colleagues who worked from home and preferred that set-up. From the outside, it might seem like a risk, allowing clients into the space where you actually live and eschewing the anonymity of hotel rooms. But in actual fact, it feels more calming because you are in your own environment and not constantly going into unfamiliar surroundings. You can assess how someone behaves in your space. Plus, living in London with full independence was my priority and this was the way to make it work financially. So I was ready to give this way of working a go. I would be doing a job that I loved with clients that I clicked well with in a beautiful part of London. I felt like I was right where I belonged.

My landlord was a very sweet man. As far as he was aware, I was a massage therapist (technically true; I had the qualifications to prove it). I had already been renting his basement flats on a short-term basis when I was toing and froing between London and Bedfordshire, so he and his staff already knew me. I had begun to build relationships and make connections with reception. I allowed them to see that I was a good person and got on their good side. My landlord didn't ask for any references or paperwork, just a deposit and rent upfront.

I felt like my new home was made for me. And, boy, did I make use of that four-poster bed! Antonio would often have me handcuffed to the railing above my head while I swayed my arse from side to side looking at myself in the mirror. It became the framework (literally) for exploring more submission, domination, bondage, tie and tease. I began to invest more into my business – toys (strap-on, rubber glove for prostate massage, blindfold, restraints), lingerie (high-end lingerie from Honey Birdette did wonders for my curves and naturally bouncy bust) and roleplay outfits (secretary, dom, latex). My spreader bar became very popular, especially with Antonio (I only used it with those I trusted). He'd have me strapped in by my ankles, legs wide apart, while he worked his magic. Within minutes he'd have me squirting into a puddle on the floor. Aside from the bar, the glove for prostate massages was my most popular investment.

I found that working for a high-end agency, the expectation and pressure to maintain a certain image increased. Once the fees began to rise, so did clients' expectations. Investing in and maintaining my image became crucial. Naturally, my overheads also began to increase. Hair appointments, personal trainers, gym memberships, tweakments, manicures, pedicures, lingerie. Plus therapist, accountant, books. And obviously the weekly essentials: condoms, lube, baby wipes, massage oils, men's body wash, men's body spray, mouthwash, Femfresh, candles. On top of the above, regular professional photos every six months were crucial. The day that new photos went up onto Archie's site bookings would soar! On my days off, I would bask in going make-up free and walking around in my comfies and flats or maxi dress and trainers in the summer. Almost like a rebellious teenager, fighting against the expectation to look a certain way.

It was the first place of my own since I was in Hampstead. I felt super protective of it. I knew what I had been through to get to that point. When I was working, I always used separate bedsheets and pillows to my own, keeping my bedding for myself. It was a good way to differentiate in my mind from work me and me me. It had a very positive psychological effect. Plus, there was no way anyone's semen or pubic hair was getting anywhere near my beautiful Egyptian cotton bedsheets and duck-down duvet! It did mean that there was mountains and mountains of washing to do every week – blankets, bed sheets, pillowcases, towels. I was scrupulous with the cleaning, the scrubbing, the bleaching, the mopping. Plus, my weekly cleansing ritual: smudging a sage stick around my apartment and cleansing out any negative energy. It worked wonders after the end of a busy week. Once my working week ended, usually around 8 p.m. on a Friday, I'd take a shower, do a count-up, crank up the music, strip the bed, empty the bins, bleach the bathroom, vacuum, put a load of washing on, then get my sage stick out and cleanse the energy.

I'd begin most mornings by blasting out my music and having a dance. Music had always been the thing that got me out of bed, ever since I was a teenager. Dancing and connecting with my body became a natural part of my morning routine. It created a positive force of energy around me. From dancing and singing, I'd then meditate, write in my gratitude journal and send love to people who had been bugging me. It worked wonders for the mind and was a great way to set up the day. Some mornings, I'd head to the gym for a training session. Other days, I'd go for a walk around the parks and connect with nature.

• • •

Shortly before moving to west London, I'd decided to take a trip back to Australia. My bestie Gemma had three small children and I wanted to go and spend time with her and help her out. I got the sense that she was feeling the pressure of motherhood and I wanted to be there to support her.

I saw that there was an offer on for the London to Dubai leg of the flight so grabbed the opportunity with both hands and upgraded to business class. My first time. I'd been pouring my heart and soul into my job, working my cotton socks off. I hadn't been on holiday for years. Not that this was your typical beach holiday in a hotel. And it was winter in Aus. But still, I felt the need to reward myself. It was amazing! I was treated like a queen: champagne, espresso martinis, cutlery and crockery, mattress, blanket, first to board, first off, smiles all around. I even treated myself to a mile-high orgasm while sprawled out in my business-class bed snuggled underneath my blanket. It was just too easy.

I landed in Australia to discover that the headline news was that a sex worker had been stabbed to death. *Of all the days*, I thought. Stabbings in Sydney were extremely rare, almost unheard of when I lived there.

Gemma did not know that I was a sex worker. When we had been friends in Sydney in the early days, I'd told her about working in erotic massage and she'd outed me to a friend. But we were older now and I was hoping to be able to tell her the truth.

I spent my first night and the next day at the Four Seasons hotel, which was heaven. I sat on the window seat of my hotel room gazing out over the city for hours. It all felt so surreal to be back. Back to where it all began. Bright blue skies and sunshine dominated the sky. The next day, I headed to Gemma's to stay for the remainder of my 'holiday'. I waited on her front porch for her to arrive home. She pulled up and I ran straight over to her. We held each other tightly and cried our eyes out with sheer joy at finally seeing each other again after years apart. I was totally smitten with her children. I felt so much love from them. It was the warmest of welcomes.

I didn't pick the most perfect time to tell her about my profession (but then again, there never is a perfect time; it has always felt like a huge risk). I think I probably began talking in too much detail, jabbering with jet leg. I don't even remember exactly how I told her or what was said. I just remember showing her Archie's website and my profile as she took it all in. There wasn't a strong reaction, more,

'Lizzie, you've been doing this for a while!' in a disapproving tone. Whether she disapproved that I'd taken so long to tell her or of the job itself I was unsure in that moment.

Things seemed OK at first but over the course of my stay, the cracks began to show, and it was clear that she had an issue with it. 'I'm just worried about your mental health doing a job like that.' And there it was, the first in a series of prejudices (or unconscious bias, or assumptions at the very least). Yet there she was, a struggling mother of three young children, in desperate need of a helping hand, losing her identity along the way, and *she* was worried about *my* mental health? I tried to make her understand that I had never been happier. I had financial freedom, independence to live my life in whichever way I chose. I loved my work and my regular clients and I loved being in London. But that's the assumption about sex workers, isn't it? That we are all mentally unwell and/or feeding a drug habit? I just found it so condescending. Gemma was exhausted, though; I could see it in her eyes.

Gemma's association with sex work was all negative. It became the elephant in the room. It wasn't so much about what was said, it was more about what was left unsaid. Gemma and I began to debate about the sex worker who had been stabbed to death. One of the headlines read: 'Stabbing victim funded extravagant travels as a sex worker'.[7] The headlines were defining Michaela Dunn by her profession and lifestyle. The article then went on to list all of the places she had been on holiday. What the hell did it matter where she went on holiday? She was murdered! The tone of the majority of news articles were very much 'well, she deserved it, she was a sex worker'. No. She did not 'deserve it'.

I was pleased to see that a fellow sex worker had written an article on the matter. It was so relevant and really struck a chord with me: 'Sex work isn't dangerous, aggressive men are dangerous' was the crux of her argument. I couldn't have agreed more. There have been plenty of stabbings of people who worked in other professions, but did the headlines define them by their profession and lifestyle? No, they did not. The article referred to the tragic killings in a café in 2014. One person who was killed had been a barrister and the other was a manager at the establishment. The city centre became a shrine filled with flowers and cards. A totally different reaction to that of the murder of the sex worker. Were their jobs to be blamed for the killings? Absolutely not. The aggressive man was.

Sex work comes with risks, yes. I am very aware of that. I am not trying to sugar-coat it. But opening my front door and stepping out into the big wide world every day, getting a taxi, going on a Tinder date, walking home at night, these also carry risks. I am sickened by the amount of CCTV footage I've seen on the news of predators carrying unconscious women, who they have just drugged, to their homes or hotels or wherever to sexually assault and rape them. Those women who were out and enjoying an evening with their friends were not the issue. The sexual predator was.

Look at what happened in Nottingham in June 2023. I cried when I heard the father of Grace O'Malley-Kumar, one of the three people stabbed at random, speaking at the memorial – 'Look after each other,' he said. I couldn't even begin to imagine their pain. Were people blaming the victims because they were students walking home at 4 a.m.? Of course not, because they were at liberty to walk home whenever they liked. Their life choices were not the issue. The aggressive man was the issue. Did Halyna Hutchins deserve to die on the set of *Rust* because she was working around guns and knew the risks? Absolutely not. And rightly so, the headlines did not blame her death on working in an environment where guns were present. She never deserved that. That was never the point in question.

The London Bridge terror attacks, the Manchester bombings and the shootings in Liverpool. None of the victims were to blame. The violent men are the problem, no matter who they target. It is no different for sex workers. It is our right to work doing a job we love and to be safe. We never, ever deserve to be at the receiving end of abuse, no matter what people say. No sex worker is ever 'asking for it' because of the job. It is the perpetrators that need to change, not the sex workers. But it's so much easier for society to blame and shame us rather than get to the root of the problem and potentially solve it because it feels better for them to put us into a box and shove us into a corner. Because sex work, even today, is *still* so stigmatised. So frowned upon. But those who stigmatise us only make us more vulnerable and empower the perpetrators. The shamers are literally helping the abusers, who know that they are more likely to get away with it because shame prevents sex workers from reporting anything.

I could tell Gemma was judging Michaela Dunn for her profession. She had the 'well, what do you expect? She was a sex worker' kind of attitude. It sickened me. At that point I began to feel alienated from her. As if I was looking at a total stranger, not my best friend from school. No matter how much we debated it, we just could not see eye to eye.

'Men talk about sex, women don't,' said Gemma one morning. Er, what? I don't think that I had ever heard such a narrow-minded statement. It triggered an argument.

I began challenging her. 'Actually, lots of women talk about sex. And guess what? It's perfectly healthy.'

We were arguing in front of the children. It was awful. I had to go outside and take a walk. It was very clear that we had grown apart. I felt like she wanted to discredit me for being a sex worker, for being sexually open and embracing who I was. In hindsight, I think my profession made her feel uncomfortable; it triggered her insecurities. She wasn't willing to learn and be curious about it with an open mind and compassion. It was all judgement and it made me feel awful.

There was clearly a whole world of stuff going on below the surface. I sensed her jealousy of my lifestyle, my independence and the financial freedom that I had worked hard to create. I felt that she was trying to punish me for the decisions that she made. God knows I made many sacrifices that were now slowly starting to pay off. I never punished my friends for having the security of a family because I always took responsibility for my decisions. I felt genuine happiness for my friends who got married and had children. But for some people, it was all too easy to point the finger and criticise the happily single, happily child-free, independent woman. And it was especially easy to point that finger when that woman was a sex worker.

Shortly after our argument, I fell sick with laryngitis and checked myself into an Airbnb. It was a strange coincidence that after telling Gemma about my job, I lost my voice. Perhaps that was nature's way of telling me something? Yet again, here was another prime example of what being honest about my profession could do. Even to friendships that went back to schooldays and had lasted for years. It really had the ability to bring out the worst in people.

My trip turned out to be the 'holiday' of affirmations. It affirmed how much I loved London, how much I loved my job and regular clients, how good I had it back in London, how I loved solitude and space to myself, how domestic, family life was not for me and how the grass was not always greener. I was literally chomping at the bit to get back to London. It was, I saw so clearly now, where my heart belonged.

• • •

Back in London, I felt very sad and let down by what was essentially the end of my friendship with Gemma. But I also felt oddly energised and focused. I had been challenged by the prejudices of a very old friend, but it hadn't shaken me – I loved my life and I knew in my heart I was doing what I wanted.

Ever the optimist and still a firm believer in the law of attraction, I knew that our friendship had wound down for good reason. It was probably lucky that I was feeling at my strongest and most confident, as not long after I got back, I had to deal with an uncomfortable situation at an outcall.

I was booked for four hours, heading to an address south of the river. In the booking notes it said 'regular client', which meant I could relax a little knowing that he was known to the agency. It was a pleasant enough journey there by cab, passing parks filled with people enjoying the summer sun having picnics and playing cricket. However, my mind was going back to one of the worst jobs I ever did at Lust – the client whose house was an absolute tip and who wanted to tickle me with feathers. At the time, I wondered why this had suddenly come up in my memory. Looking back, it was my intuition warning me.

The cab pulled up to a rundown terraced house with a black door, which was answered by a scruffy-looking man dressed in nothing but a dressing gown (just like the awful booking at Lust). His hair looked like it hadn't had a brush through it since 1963. The booking was almost identical to 'Mr Feather Man'. Then there was the house itself. Absolute filth. I walked into the lounge – on the floor was a blow-up bed covered in towels. The carpet was covered in dirt. Porn that looked like it was from the 1970s was playing on the TV. There were two glasses of champagne on the coffee table and, weirdly, a present wrapped up in Christmas paper.

I always try to see the good in people. When people ask me, 'How do you do this job?' it's always the same answer: 'As soon as I meet someone I look for the positive.' And that is pretty much my outlook on life in general. I've always been a glass-half-full kind of person. But this particular booking was an exception.

I didn't get the sense that he was a bad guy, but he was no angel, joking about locking me in the room when I wanted to go out to change into my lingerie and give him the big reveal. I didn't like that at all. It immediately got my back up. At that point, I decided there was no way I was going to drink any of his alcohol. Previous experiences had taught me it was not good to be vulnerable and out of it in front of clients. Especially new clients in unfamiliar, messy territory. I'd also heard that a colleague at Archie's had ended up in hospital after having her drink spiked by a regular. I wondered if this was that regular.

I tried and I tried but I just could not last longer than an hour. I had to get out. He gestured at me with his hands to come over to him. At this point, he hadn't touched or kissed me yet. I just couldn't do it. For the next few minutes I debated in my head what I was going to say to get me the hell out. *I could go upstairs to use the loo and say I've just come on my period, or I could just be honest and say I'm not comfortable here. Shit, fuck, I need to get out, I don't want to hurt his feelings but there is filth everywhere. Today is Saturday. I don't usually work Saturdays. I should be at home cooking in the kitchen, singing and dancing.*

In the end, I just had to say, 'I'm sorry, darling, I'm just not comfortable here. I think it's best we finish the booking and you have someone else come over. It's just the chemistry is not right for me, nothing personal. Sometimes it happens.' I made out like it was all to do with the chemistry and nothing to do with the complete shithole he was living in. All he kept saying was, 'I don't understand what I've done wrong.' Over and over I just kept assuring him that the chemistry wasn't right for me so it was best I gave him the rest of the money back and leave. I got up and wiped the dirt from my knees and began to put my clothes back on.

As soon as I got in the cab I called Archie. 'I'm sorry, Archie, but I couldn't stay any longer. The house was absolute filth. He had a blow-up bed on the floor in the lounge. I just couldn't last four hours on it. We went to go upstairs but he had no curtains and another blow-up bed on the floor.'

'He had a blow-up bed on the floor?' he said in total disbelief. 'Don't worry, darling, I'm totally with you when it comes to cleanliness. I'm surprised you managed to stay there for one hour.' I just loved how understanding he was.

I asked Archie to check the history of the client's bookings to see if anyone else had made the same complaint. He had seen one girl eighteen times but it was all incalls. And that's the difference between incalls and outcalls. I'm sure I would have been OK with this client in my own clean and tidy space, but it was too late: the damage had been done, and I didn't want to see him again. There had been previous outcalls to his home, though. Surely these ladies must have said something?

As soon as I got back to my flat I went straight to the bathroom and had a scorching-hot shower, scrubbing myself clean over and over, followed by a trip to Burger King for a bacon double cheeseburger meal. Large. To round off my whole cleansing ritual I made myself a cup of tea, thanked my lucky stars I was no longer in the house of mess and didn't touch myself for days. It's as though I had to shut that part of myself off for some time in order to recover. By the following week, it was soon forgotten about and I was back to touching myself every few days.

What a contrast that experience was to the night before, when I'd been at the ME hotel in the Strand, guzzling cocktails at the Radio Rooftop Bar on a beautiful summer's evening. This job was varied, yes, but this level of variation at Archie's was extremely rare. The 'house of mess' experience was a one-off and I have not had an experience like that since. It showed me that I was beginning to realise my own worth and to set higher standards when it came to clients. I was worth more than being in a dirty house on a blow-up bed.

However, that was not the end of the bad streak. The following Monday, I had a booking at the Hard Rock Hotel. I was greeted by a group of very drunken and unruly lads. It was just me and three of them in the room – which was intimidating, to say the least. I didn't trust that situation at all so I charged a cancellation fee and bolted.

On the odd occasion when I felt unsure about a client, it often felt safer to just leave rather than hang around waiting for a cancellation fee. This can feel like a risk. I had 'rejected' them and you never know how someone will react in that situation. Some clients used it as an opportunity to drag things out to ensure I had to stay talking to them for longer. Safety comes above everything, definitely always above money. I wasn't willing to do anything with anyone and everyone. It may have felt like I was losing out in the short term, but I was gaining so much more in the long run.

But these experiences were rare. The good absolutely outweighed the bad. It always did. I acquired more wonderful regulars at Archie's and was beginning to build quite a reputation. My list of reviews on the website was growing. These were important and always came as a welcome way to boost bookings. Straight from the horse's mouth:

As always, a wonderful, sensual and fun experience with the beautiful, lovely Olivia. We embraced together in romantic acquaintance in warm sensual grace. Lovely shining beautiful eyes and of course that smile. That glowing, beautiful smile.

She caressed my feet and whispered something incredibly naughty in my ear which caused me to look up at her and say yes madam I'll do anything you say. After we embarked on the usual naughtiness, she began to tell me a story about my fantasy and had remembered everything from years back. I kneeled in front of the altar and caressed and worshipped in awe.

Olivia, you are the best best friend, the best lover. The best person to understand the sequence of my mind to express with the words of love and care. You leave me with memories of your intense sexuality and beauty. Which will hold me for many many months to come before I have the opportunity to see you again.

Of course, it's an ego boost to get a great review from a client enthusing about how hot you are, how much you turned them on, etc. Who wouldn't enjoy that, right?! But really, when I look back over the course of my career, it's the people who have said to me, 'Thank you, I feel better,' that I remember with pride. 'Coming to see you is like my therapy. You are my doctor!' said Dinesh one happy, sunny lunchtime.

'You are my therapy too – we help each other,' I assured him. We embraced and held each other just for a moment before he left grinning like the Chesire cat.

Another regular client was such a lovely, kind-hearted soul. After one booking, just before he left, he turned to me and said, 'I was having a really bad day and feeling really low but now I feel so much better after seeing you. My brother died three years ago today.' I gave him the biggest hug and hoped my warm embrace remained with him for the rest of the day. Comments like these made the job worth it. And hence why I felt more like a therapist than a sex worker. The profession really does help people in more ways than outsiders realise. It all goes back to human connection. The desire for skin-on-skin contact. Sometimes that comes in the form of mind-blowing sexual chemistry, and other times it comes in the form of conversation, of being held and being listened to.

• • •

I'd been having an average day. Nothing too memorable, just bookings with clients that I didn't click particularly well with. So I didn't have high hopes for the next client that was due any minute. When I opened the door, I was pleasantly surprised. Richard was a very handsome man, all smiles, cleanshaven, very friendly. Immediately I felt a huge sense of relief from his energy. My whole body relaxed so I knew I was in for a good time. We chatted, we engaged, we clicked almost instantly.

My intuition was right about Richard from the get-go. He became undoubtedly my most reliable and loyal client for many years. It amazes me how we've grown together sexually over all the years that we've known each other. Richard was one of the few clients who would religiously book me around the same time once a month, every month, without fail for years. Over time, we began to build trust not just sexually, but also in opening up about our personal lives. I saw him as a very good friend with whom I had mind-blowing sex. With whom I felt confident exploring different parts of myself. I helped him tap into his dominant side and he did the same for me. I always knew that I could fully relax when Richard was on his way. More like a friend popping over.

We'd always start the booking with a quick chat and catch-up, which was always a good way of setting the tone. As we matured, so did our sexual exploration. Every single time it would be fireworks and it would baffle us both how it just seemed to get better and better as time progressed. I would love to have got to the point where I could only allow space for regular clients. Regular clients were my bread and butter.

Raj was a tall, gentle man. We partied a lot together but on the other hand we'd often share stories and read our poems to each other. We created a space that felt safe for us to both be vulnerable together. I developed a soft spot for him and began to grow more and more concerned for him as I could see his drug and alcohol use spiral out of control. He told me that he was unhappy in his marriage but refused to get a divorce because of his children. Presumably his reliance on drugs and alcohol was related to this. It got to the point where his dealer refused to sell him more cocaine. Hats off to the dealer.

This was an all too familiar scene, largely among men in their fifties. And, on that note, I'm not prepared to take responsibility for someone else's infidelity. That is their wrongdoing, not mine. I support women as much as I can given my situation; teaching clients how to properly pleasure a woman, how to be respectful and highlighting the fact that women also have sexual needs. In rare instances where clients have appeared arrogant and cocky, I have soon put them in their place by assuring them that their partner more than likely knows about their infidelity and is most probably having some fun of their own. Their expression soon changes.

But, yet again, it is so much easier to point the finger at the woman, especially when that woman is a sex worker. That's the easy option. We are just doing our job. Half the time, we don't even know what a client's relationship status is. It's rarely talked about. And, even so, I'm not here to judge anyone. If it wasn't me, it would be someone else. Would you blame a bartender for serving alcohol unknowingly to a recovering alcoholic? The bartender is just doing their job. It is up to the individual to own their actions and take responsibility. Abusive behaviour towards sex workers because of someone else's infidelity is not only wrong, but not beneficial to anyone and does not get to the root of the issue. Some clients have told me that their partner gave them their blessing to see a sex worker and specifically picked me out. Every situation is different. Life is not a one-size-fits-all scenario.

Around this time, I read an article about how middle-aged men were almost forgotten about, yet suicide rates among them were some of the highest of all age groups. The headline read: 'We are shamefully ignoring the plight of middle-aged men'. With so much focus being on the younger generation, who are grappling with their own mental health issues growing up in the shadow of the climate crisis, with all the complications social media brings, it's easy to overlook men in their forties and fifties. A lot of these men were well-off, successful at work and ostensibly very privileged. But still, often I felt more like a therapist. I am not a qualified therapist, of course, so with clients like Raj there was only so much I could do, but I was at least able to get him to open up and talk more about his emotions, and help to reassure and comfort him. A lot of sex workers do genuinely care, especially about regular clients with whom we have built a connection.

• • •

I was really enjoying the balance of incalls and outcalls. Dinner dates and trips to the casinos and hotels were great opportunities to get out and about in the jungle. There was certainly something quite freeing about going out to work rather than clients coming to my home all the time, although I did now have my apartment set up perfectly and I was still so happy to have my own space. My video intercom was a great addition. About five minutes before a client's arrival, I'd stand and watch. When a new client arrived at my door, I had a moment to observe their movements, their mannerisms, their physicality, their energy.

Of course there were some days when I struggled to get motivated. Just like with any job. It would usually be during either a summer heatwave or in the thick of winter when it felt like the whole world was in hibernation and I wanted nothing more than to be snuggled on the couch, candles glowing all around me, rain banging down on the window, comfies on with a cup of tea and a good book. Occasionally, during quieter periods, I'd be all set up for an evening in my own company and get the shock of my life to receive a last-minute booking with twenty minutes' notice to get ready! I'd then have to somehow transform from the 'snuggled on the couch' version of me to the 'fantasy-like creature' version of me …

In the early days, I would panic and text Archie straight away: 'Archie, I can't be ready in twenty minutes, I need more time!'

'OK darling, we'll see if the client can push back ten minutes.' The key for achieving the transformation at short notice was always music. I'd put the right playlist on, jump up and get organised. Then, more often than not, the extra ten minutes was fine. But it still meant I only had half an hour to totally transform not just physically, but also mentally, and some days it felt like a push.

More recently, I have learnt to take it all in my stride. I've got pretty good at turning things around very quickly. Make-up and hair I can usually do in fifteen minutes. One thing the job has taught me is to take the bloody pressure off, to have confidence in myself. With no disrespect to men, this job has taught me how 'simple' men's expectations are, especially compared to those that I put on myself. They are just happy to see a bright and bubbly curvaceous blonde with a bit of lippy on. On days when I've felt like I don't look my best, clients have showered me with compliments. I might have been due on my period, felt horrendously bloated and struggled to squeeze myself into my lingerie and yet clients have left grinning from ear to ear – 'That was amazing, Olivia. I will definitely be back!'

This has been a very useful lesson about the crazy amount of pressure us ladies put on ourselves. Not just sex workers, but women everywhere. The rise of social media and filters has not helped as it has created an unobtainable idea of perfection, of being flawless.

A hugely positive thing that the job has taught me is that no one else is scrutinising my body in the way I have scrutinised myself. As I've got older and more experienced, I increasingly feel able to own who I am, be proud of my curves and not apologise for being anything other than me. Men love all body shapes, natural curves as well as athletic body types. There is something out there for everyone. I have realised it all comes back to energy again. Greeting clients with a big smile and upbeat energy helped to get bookings off to a flying start. *That's* what people are drawn to.

Only a couple of times throughout my career has a client tried to shame me for my curves. As one client came through the door, he looked me up and down, nipped at my stomach and said, 'Sorry, too much of a belly for me!' and walked out of the door. Charming! I got the impression that it wasn't the first time he had done this – perhaps he even got off on trying to bring sex workers down. Slightly ironically, he was a dishevelled, unattractive old man who did not take care of himself at all, so I was grateful he left. Needless to say, he went straight onto my banned list. Another time, I was fully dressed in my lingerie, with my silk dressing gown wrapped around my goods, heels on. The client walked in and asked to take a look. I obliged and undid my robe. 'No, sorry,' he said and walked out of the door. *Thank God*, I thought. He was not my type at all and his energy stank. I do not need these clients anywhere near me. My regulars adored my natural curves – 'Now that's a body!' Mr Dom once said as he stood behind me whispering into my ear, hands manoeuvring all over my bottom.

My trusted regular Charlie had no issues with me being in my pyjamas; sometimes he'd even insist. I think Charlie would have been happy if I answered the door wearing nothing but a bin bag. My style began to centre very much around the 1950s with my own modern twist. Classic black Christian Louboutins (the only designer item I have ever purchased). Lots of knee-length pencil dresses and skirts, office wear. Fitted bodysuits to accentuate my curves. Tailored trousers from Zara. Lots of trench coats, lots of black. My black Karen Millen jumpsuit highlighted my curves perfectly, though it was a tight fit; while at a dinner date with a client at Murano in Mayfair, I had to stick my head around the bathroom door and signal to him that I needed help getting in and out of it. He soon got out of his chair, more than happy to oblige.

I have built up my collection of Honey Birdette pieces over the years – red lace, white lace, baby-blue corsets, black bondage, lots and lots of stockings. Red and black has always worked best for me. Classic colours. Along with my shiny, manicured red nails.

I love my food – food and sex, to me, are the natural pleasures of life. I'd much rather go food shopping than clothes shopping. A nice long lunch with friends is one of my favourite ways to spend an afternoon. However, when I am on shift I am careful about what I eat as I don't want to eat a big dinner and then feel sluggish and bloated afterwards. This job requires energy at the best of times! On my days off, however, I'd be straight in the kitchen to cook up a storm or heading out for dinner with friends.

I have been on some very enjoyable dinner dates with clients to some incredible restaurants, but I am at work, so to an extent I am playing the character of Olivia. It's my job to maintain the fantasy. So (unless I'm out with Charlie; there's always an exception to the rule) it's not the same as being in a restaurant with friends where I can relax and be my unguarded self. Overnight bookings can come with similar challenges. I'm playing a part and can't fully let go and be myself – even when I'm asleep! It's basically an acting job that lasts all through the night. Also, I think most people are familiar with the slight awkwardness that can come with waking up with someone you don't know that well. You're conscious of the morning breath, the morning gas and maybe the need for a morning poop. Well, sex workers have all of that too – we are only human!

I have definitely been in the position of clenching my butt cheeks together as hard as I could while we lay in bed together, following a three- or four-course meal the night before with lashings of alcohol! Before the human reality of Olivia was revealed, I'd freshen up, say my goodbyes and make a swift exit. Or tactfully hustle the client out of the door.

Working as a high-end sex worker in west London gave me a nice lifestyle. The money I was making meant I could spoil my friends and family. I could pay for meals and buy nice gifts for birthdays, which I absolutely love to do. I surprised Freddie by putting some money in his account for his holiday. I hadn't forgotten the time when I was broke and he had helped me out. It felt so good to be able to treat and help out others now. Especially a unique friend like Freddie. For myself, I was never huge on shopping or designer labels; spoiling myself was all about good food and massage treatments. (If I could live anywhere, I'd live in a spa!) However, probably the most important aspect of my job is the freedom it gives me.

From previous experience, I know only too well that working the monotonous nine-to-five in an office environment is just not me. I never lost that need to head out on my own adventure that I had as a child on the farm. I have always valued time alone to restore myself and being a sex worker allows this. I only needed to be working three or four days a week at a pace that worked for me. The rest of the time I could recharge, see friends and commit time to volunteering. I spent two hours a week as a 'befriender' to someone who was struggling mentally. We'd go for walks, brunch or visit galleries. It was a wonderful experience and I am so glad my job afforded me the time to do it. It was the icing on the cake when I heard from the charity that the person who I had spent time with had told them that I had made a big positive difference to their life.

• • •

When it comes to roleplay, most sex workers are happy to oblige. It does take a certain amount of imagination and focus, but that's all part of the fun! Having obtained a master's in acting, it is something I have always found quite easy. Despite it being a huge cliché, 'sexy secretary' is the perennial favourite that I don't think will ever go away. Whether it's something to do with increasingly higher standards for appropriate behaviour in workplaces making it feel more taboo – and therefore more sexy – or if it's just such a staple storyline in porn that young men internalise it at a young age, I have no idea. All I can say is that I have donned a pair of glasses and been bent over 'the boss's desk' more times than I can count. The others that come up regularly are massage therapist/client ('Oh, I'm sorry, sir, my hand slipped!'), tenant/landlord, property owner/ cleaner and, interestingly, quite a few want me to pretend to be the girlfriend of their best friend.

Much to my delight, Antonio began to book more regularly, sometimes twice a week. I always looked forward to bookings with him as I knew I would be in for a good time. We explored more and more with different kinds of roleplay. One morning, he had me scrubbing and cleaning my flat, pretending I was doing a 'trial run' for a cleaning job. He was the potential employer, I was the cleaner. This was my kind of roleplay. *Two-in-one job today*, I thought to myself. *I'm getting paid to clean my own flat. Win win!*

However, the issue with Antonio was that the more time we spent together, the more I felt connected to him, and feelings were starting to develop. *Uh oh*, I thought. *I've been here before, I know how horribly this can end. This is not good.* One day, a colleague told me that he had booked her and I was surprised at how much it hurt. But really, what did I expect? I had learnt many times over what falling for clients leads to. However, after some time apart I was able to move on from it all and continue to see Antonio for many years after. Now there are no feelings at all. It's purely physical.

I think all the drugs and partying were having a huge influence on my wellbeing at that time. Inevitably, they blurred my sense of reality and I was starting to grow more and more tired of it. It had got to a point where, after partying with clients, once they had left, I'd often continue partying and doing drugs on my own, dancing in my room listening to music until the early hours. That's when I knew I had a problem. Especially the next day when I was unable to face anyone or anything, and I found myself cancelling bookings and hiding in my bedroom all day ordering junk food. *I hate this*, I always thought when I'd got myself in this state.

I was partying and doing drugs long before I began working as a sex worker. I had always been a total hedonist. I would have hunted the drugs and alcohol down whatever job I'd ended up doing. But I was beginning to realise that I didn't want to be living that lifestyle anymore. It took away everything that was positive about me. The more alcohol I drank and the more drugs I took, the more frustrated I got with myself. I began to see myself more and more as a businesswoman and started looking into ways that I could use my experiences as a sex worker to make life better for others.

Contrary to popular belief, there is nothing glamorous about cocaine – heart palpitations, paranoia, anxiety, panic attacks, fucked-up stomach, snotty nose and living in constant fear of shitting myself (snorting a product laced with baby laxative tends to do that) were not in the least bit sexy. It really is the 'arsehole's' drug in its ability to bring out the worst in people. I also began to hate how vulnerable I made myself after drinking alcohol. I never made any good decisions when drinking and people, mostly when I socialised outside of work, took advantage. I am friendly and chatty at the best of times, but alcohol made me far too friendly for my liking.

A new me was beginning to emerge. I was slowly starting to turn my focus in a new direction and onto a healthier path. I realised that I had got to the point where I was just doing drugs for the sake of it, because they were there, because clients had them, not because I wanted to. I was growing sick and tired of that whole cycle. The comedowns were becoming unbearable. I didn't know how or when, but I knew deep down that I was getting closer and closer to hitting the partying lifestyle on the head. I knew it was going to take some time to undo almost twenty years of habits. That wasn't going to happen overnight. I knew that I had to take the view that this would be a process if I were to give up the drugs and alcohol for good. And a big part of that would involve cleansing out any friends who did drugs and partied with me. I had to cut myself off from all associations if I were to ever live a healthier lifestyle.

A new woman was being born – a strong, assertive, business-minded woman. Finally, I'd had enough of the partying days, getting wrecked and feeling like crap the next day. I was now ready to challenge myself and pursue my goals. It became more and more important to me to stay focused, to meditate and to distance myself from toxic people.

• • •

Around this time, I decided to make a move to work independently. I had heard a lot about independent sites from colleagues. Not having to pay a commission to agencies and being able to keep 100 per cent of my earnings sounded very appealing, as did being fully in charge of my own schedule and having direct communication with clients, with no 'middleman' reception desk to occasionally miscommunicate or mix up messages. There was no issue with Archie's; I had loved working for him. I had just heard so much about working independently and fancied a change. I rang Archie and was very open and honest with him. I think he was surprised but understood, though he did warn me that a lot of clients who were banned from agencies ended up on the independent sites. No matter what job I've done, I've always felt it best to leave on a positive note. Be professional and charming to the very end. Because you never know which direction life will take you, and if ever you'll need to return. I found it beneficial to keep many baskets open to many eggs.

My early opinion of working through an independent site was that it was a bit hit and miss, and very much like shopping in the sales. Every now and then I'd find a little gem. The website I was using was a bit too tacky for my liking but I did like the freedom that came with it. The review system that underpinned it was very beneficial to both client and sex worker. If a potential client had any bad reviews, it was just a no from me. It wasn't worth the risk. A few of my clients from Archie's tracked me down, which I was very pleased to see.

One evening, I had a last-minute dinner-date request come through for two guys. They wanted two ladies so I invited a colleague who I used to work with at Archie's. Frankie was by far the best duo buddy. We had great chemistry and we had a lot of fun together on our adventures as sex workers. Once, after a night of partying at my place, I woke to find a ginormous double-ended dildo in my kitchen sink. *Geez, what the hell happened last night? Must have been a good night!* I thought to myself. I texted Frankie: 'You left your dildo at mine. I'll drop it off next time I pop round.'

We met the clients at the Ivy. They were easy-going, cheeky and fun. One super sexy, one not so. I went with the smoking-hot one. Again, that night proved that good looks don't always equal the best bookings. He had me crawling around his hotel room floor on a leash like some kind of pet. I was beginning to grow tired of being submissive. I felt like the dominant within me was growing stronger and stronger and beginning to find her own voice.

I was also on a roll with my savings, gaining more and more momentum. More regulars and more repeat bookings. After a morning gym session, I sat down in the changing rooms to take a moment and check my bank balance. My savings were finally in the five figures. I looked up, thanking the universe with a huge sense of relief. My time in the industry was starting to pay off. I was getting closer and closer to getting on that property ladder.

ELIZABETH G.

It was through the independent site that I met Christopher – an absolute diamond in a sea of hits and misses. He was incredibly sensual and so wonderfully giving. The first time we met, he insisted on massaging me, which hadn't happened in a long time. It was very rare that a client offered to do this but always very welcome. It was one of those 'I can't believe I'm getting paid to do this' kind of moments. The more giving a client is with me, the more giving I am in return. It's a two-way street.

Christopher began to book me on a regular basis. We'd sometimes meet out for dinner, at a bar or even my local pub, to start the booking. With him it was easy: conversation flowed, we clicked and had insane sexual chemistry. He'd always come fully stocked with candles. Once back at my place, the room would be glowing with candlelight as he doused my body in oil, teasing the crap out of me, our bodies slipping and sliding in total sensual bliss. Heaven! We even shared a love of sporting events. When the football was on, we'd either go to the pub and get involved with the crowds or set up at mine. I'd provide the drinks and nibbles. He was a total joy to be around and exactly the type of client I wanted to attract. No blurred lines, no trying to seduce me, just very clear cut. We both knew where we stood with each other. That was exactly how I liked it. I was happy with the way we were around each other and thought my days of falling for clients were well behind me. But, as they say, pride comes before a fall.

CHAPTER TEN
LESSONS

I was not blown away by Mr M – he was just another unhappy, middle-aged man having a midlife crisis, I thought. He was well dressed, polite, clean, well groomed, respectful and friendly. All the things that a sex worker looks for in a client. But other than that, he was just a client. End of. He made no lasting impression on me. When he left after our first meeting, he was gone from my mind and my life continued.

After only a couple of meetings, he invited me out to dinner. I was very pleased as I had been going through a bit of a dry spell with dinner dates, so this was a welcome surprise. I needed the cash, yes, but I was pleased that I was going to be taken out for the first time in what felt like forever, after a period when it felt like a lot of men just wanted sex and drugs from me. Little did I know where Mr M's head was at; I just thought he wanted a chat over dinner.

As I stepped out of my building feeling oh so glam in my black leather knee-length pencil skirt, red shirt and shiny stilettos, I got my heel caught in the mat on the doorstep. There went the illusion of effortless glamour! I noticed a man standing on the pavement staring directly at me. Fixated. I was without my glasses, so his face was a bit of a blur. Then I realised it was Mr M. He came straight to my assistance and lifted my heel out of the mat like a perfect gentleman. It was only after our third meeting that the first red flag came my way. A red flag I chose to ignore.

ELIZABETH G.

Dearest Olivia,

Our time together over the last few weeks has all been quite remarkable. I accept that my perspective on our connection will be different to yours, nonetheless I appreciate we both seem to feel a strong connection with each other and so far as I see it that is a really good thing.

With that in mind, I want to tell you that you are the sort of lady I am deeply attracted to – beautiful, intelligent, sensual and honest. No doubt there are facets to your personality I have not seen so far, all the same those which I have seen are strongly attractive. Maybe there is no need to tell you that at a primal level I find you deeply physically attractive; there is so much more. I felt quite comfortable talking over dinner, and am eager to know more about you. I have nothing to hide from you, and want to share my world with you.

I have no expectations or demands, so while I have gut instinct desire and wishes which over time may play out, I need you to know that I have no intention of exerting any control or restriction on who you are, who you see, what you do or when you do it. You are a brilliant woman, I have no desire, wish or intention to distract from this at any time. You may reasonably and sensibly feel that I am coming on too strong and too heavily; it is in your gift to let me know.

You are a beautiful woman, you fill me with turbulent emotions, thank you. xxx.

I was totally flabbergasted. We had only met a few times prior to him sending me this message. I should have known there and then: coming on strong early on is a clear warning. It was right there in the message: 'No agenda/no intention/I have nothing to hide from you/I'm not this, not that, etc., etc.' – when someone feels they have to insist that they aren't possessive, hiding anything or harbouring negative intentions from the get-go, more often than not, they are. That is a warning to sign to get the hell out of there. They are testing the waters and giving you a preview of what is to come. I don't stalk people so I don't need to mention when I first meet someone, 'I won't stalk you.' In fact, Mr M even said very early on: 'Don't worry, I won't start stalking you.' At the time I just laughed it off and didn't think much of it.

I responded, trying to play down his over-the-top, long-winded message:

Thank you for your message. Wow, I don't really know where to start. It does feel really great to have such a strong connection with you and I loved our time together last night. It's been so long since I have been treated like that and it made me feel very special indeed.

I think it's really great that we are both clearly attracted to each other and I'm excited to see where this leads. It's very early days of course and I like to take things slow. And you already figured out that I do have my guard up, which I don't let down very easily. It's largely based on past experiences and really to protect myself. I really do love your company and find you incredibly attractive so let's live in the moment and enjoy each other xx

I really should have known there and then that something was up. In fact, at this point I had already seen the ten-year review history on his profile. Ten years?! That was one of the longest review histories I had ever seen. He had been visiting sex workers regularly for a decade. It was clearly a big part of his life. I noticed that on one occasion he had gone back to the same sex worker twice in a day. Something didn't sit right. I didn't hold back and made my feelings known to him: 'I am on to you,' I playfully warned him as I waved my finger at him while we were drinking in my local.

A risk with going independent was that I didn't have the umbrella of protection that I got from working with an agency. I was managing my own bookings and clients had a direct line to me, including Mr M, of course. Some felt entitled to message me any time of day, even late at night or in the middle of the night, as if they expected me to be available for a chat 24/7. You wouldn't do that to your doctor, lawyer or therapist, would you? I personally wouldn't – that would be disrespecting their boundaries.

I overlooked the red flags mostly because, from the very beginning, Mr M was so incredibly charming – a smooth talker a great listener, so curious about me and so full of flattery. For the first time in a long time, I felt truly 'seen' and the apple of a man's eye. Still, at this point, I remained guarded. I knew only too well where falling for clients got me. After Shaun, and a few flings in between, I had a wall of steel securely built around me. Or so I thought. I was not prepared for what was to come next.

We initially connected over our love of fast cars, country life and country pursuits. We were both very sensual and sexually open. We'd spend hours chatting at dinner in glitzy west-London restaurants, having deep and meaningful conversations, eyes fixed on each other as though time stood still. He was even able to give me some much-needed business advice and guidance for my side projects. It was beginning to feel like a real partnership. A relationship.

It didn't take long for me to be smitten. Despite everything I'd told myself about not falling for clients, despite my previous experiences, I fell. Hard. Mr M was loving, kind, giving, intuitive to my needs and my body. He had a willingness to learn about me. He listened and I totally believed that he cared. Plus he was handsome, well dressed and intelligent. We became inseparable.

Over and over, he painted a picture of an amazing future for us. One that I wanted so much. His certainty and his charm smashed down any protective barrier I put up. I no longer thought of him as a client. I was in love.

One evening, we went out for dinner in Kensington. We were fixated on each other all night, laughed our heads off, then went back to mine and made love. I had one of the most powerful orgasms I'd ever had. The next morning, we went out for breakfast. The rain was beating down around us while we were surrounded by the warm glow of fairy lights. Absorbing each other, learning about each other.

The love I felt was so incredibly powerful, like a force I had never felt before. I had no doubt in my mind that Mr M was the man I wanted to spend the rest of my life with. I never felt such strong love to the point where I was terrified at the thought of losing him. We were living in a dream. Not reality.

Maybe it was because Mr M seemed so different from Shaun that I failed to take proper heed of the warning signs. He was a lot older, for a start, in his early fifties. An old-school gentleman with a soothing energy, he was a completely different character to the 'geezer' that was Shaun. Also, he didn't do drugs – which was what I so desperately needed at the time. It didn't even occur to me to compare the two of them, to notice the similarities in the beginning of the relationship.

However, another major red flag soon appeared. He had told me that he was separated and living apart from his ex, co-parenting their daughter. It sounded complicated so initially I was cautious. Particularly as he had seemed reluctant to give anything about himself away. My intuition was telling me that something about this man felt a little off but, unusually, I didn't listen. He told me again and again that he and his ex were waiting for their daughter to turn eighteen before they began divorce proceedings, until I truly believed it.

I told Mr M about what had happened with Shaun. A major error, I now see, but I was reassured by how shocked and supportive he was about that whole ordeal. He in turn began to share and open up about his own traumas. He may have been sketchy on the details of his life away from me but the fact that he was being honest about his feelings and vulnerabilities masked that and made me think I knew him. The connection felt unbelievable.

The texts and emails came thick and fast. 'You mean the world to me.' 'I love you.' 'I want to touch you, to hold you and to reassure you of my feelings.' 'We have decades of love ahead of us.'

We began to build on what was starting to feel like a solid and secure relationship. But as time progressed and we grew closer and fell even more in love, out of nowhere, he would cut me out cold. Nothing. He would disappear for weeks. Sometimes ghost me. I was beside myself. He was my partner, my lover. I had believed everything he had said. He declared his undying love for me and had me planning our lives together one minute, then dropped me like a ton of bricks, cutting all communication and telling me that he could never see me again the next. This became a pattern of behaviour that played out over the best part of a year and started to feel like madness on repeat.

In these times I would berate myself. What did I expect? He was a client. I was a sex worker. How could I have been so stupid to allow a client to relentlessly burrow his way into my heart, after everything I went through with Shaun? I was heartbroken and bereft. During these times of sorrow, I resolved to pick myself up and carry on. That was always the moment when he would push his way back into my life.

It's hard to put into words in a way that makes sense to someone who has never been in this position just how ceaselessly, how persistently, he pursued me, and the level of emotional manipulation he put me under. We would have the most blazing rows – there were scenes in restaurants, scuffles in my hallway and once he called me 'a cheap fucking whore', just as Shaun had done. I would decide it was over, there was no way I was going back there again. But then the messages would start:

I realise that I have overstepped the mark, I put you in a position and I am wholly responsible for the situation you are in. Your health and happiness is all that really matters, you are a strong and independent woman, a beautiful and creative woman. Could you please let me know you are safe? Despite everything, you mean the world to me and I am worried. If you would like to speak, I shall be available all day today.

He would blame himself, grovel, apologise and pull on my heartstrings:

I know my actions are my responsibility, I know that I destroyed our relationship. I cannot tell you what drove me to be so mean and nasty. I have a self-destruct button hard wired in me which I press when good things start to happen in my life, you are well aware of that. Waking today I am hollow, I want to touch you, to be held by you and feel safe like I felt when I was in your company. I've not ever recognised that before, but I did feel safe when I was with you.

I've fucked up everything good in my life, I'm so sorry my fuck up has impacted on you – your instincts were right. So sorry. You are an exceptional woman, you will meet an exceptional partner and be truly happy very soon.

He would stop at nothing to worm his way back into my heart. It was all made worse because, by this time, we were living through a global pandemic and a series of lockdowns. It magnified the hurt by a thousand. It was mental torture for my sensitive soul.

At the start of the first lockdown, I had been determined to stay in London. I didn't want to run away from my beloved west London at the first sign of panic. I wanted to still feel the energy of people around me, not isolate myself even further at my parents' farm. My landlord also slashed my rent in half, which I was hugely grateful for. I had worked so hard for that flat, I was not going to give it up without a fight. I had my self-employment grants from the government to live off. *Honesty really does pay off*, I thought, pleased that all my finances were totally above board and I had declared my income from the very beginning because it made me eligible for a grant that helped me to survive through a pandemic.

But, like so many of us at that time, I was lonely. And I missed Mr M with a physical ache. I began to hate the evenings as that was when I longed for human interaction the most. Just simple things like meeting a friend for dinner or going to my local pub. I began to feel the frustration of lockdown and limited movement. The social butterfly within me was feeling trapped and I was dying to be out on a dance floor losing myself. I dreaded going to bed, facing another sleepless night.

In the first lockdown, Mr M was at home in the countryside with his 'ex-wife' and daughter. That was the only way they could both see her, he said. It was killing me but I knew there was no other option – that was where he had to be.

As time progressed, however, more hidden truths came out. It turned out he hadn't ever been living separately to his 'ex-wife', as he had repeatedly told me. They were separated but still living together, sleeping in separate bedrooms while co-parenting their daughter, was the revised version of the story. It hurt. But I'd heard it before – couples who were no longer together but still living together in separate rooms while they figured out an alternative arrangement. In this modern day, it wasn't unusual. *It will be OK*, I told myself. We just need to see each other again.

• • •

But when we did see each other again, we had another major argument. On this particular instance I'd discovered that he was not separated from his wife at all. Was everything he said a lie? This time it was over, I was sure. I loved this man like I had never loved anyone but I couldn't cope with the hurt or the headfuck anymore. I had to get him out of my life for good. I blocked his number and his email. I was determined to move on.

I had come to see more clearly that there had been other factors that had left me open to his relentless pursuit of me, had made me ignore my instincts and close my eyes to the red flags. I had grown tired of all the drugs and partying but I hadn't yet got to the point where I could figure out how to meaningfully change my lifestyle. It was burning me out. The fact that Mr M didn't do drugs had, ironically, given me the impression that he would be 'healthier' for me. There was also the money. At the beginning, he had offered a monthly payment. This felt less transactional than it usually did with clients because the money just went into my account once a month without me thinking about it. This payment had helped keep me afloat during the uncertainty of Covid, which perhaps subconsciously made me see him as someone to be relied on. But that was, of course, just money. It guaranteed nothing at all but temporary financial security. And perhaps those wounds from Shaun were not as healed as I thought they were. Mr M knew about what had happened with Shaun. He found a weak spot and made his move.

Heartbroken, I tried my best to carve out some space in my life that was just for me. Something to hold on to as I came to terms with the end of this insanely tumultuous relationship. I decided to reconnect with my country roots and begin riding again. Only about a forty-five-minute drive from my place in west London, I began loaning an ex-racehorse called Chester. It became my absolute solace and saving grace. It was something positive that I could put my energy into, it gave me a focus for the day. As with many, nature helped me through the pandemic: riding through woodland, and walks in Hyde Park with my friend Pippa, whom I had met the previous year while volunteering. I lived in my gym gear, riding gear and pyjamas.

But then, the day before New Year's Eve 2020, I had a riding accident. During the winter months, the horses at the yard were all locked in their stables and not turned out into the fields during the day. I didn't agree with this personally. When I was growing up on the farm, we let the horses out in the fields come rain or shine, even snow. They are large, powerful animals that need that time outside to buck and rear, to feel the open space around them. To feel their true wild and free selves. I could relate. The Covid restrictions added to this mounting pressure. There were obviously no competitions on, no going to the gallops or cross-country fields for training. It showed. I could see it in the horses, their pent-up energy, their frustration. Lockdown was getting to them too. One of the women at the yard got bucked off and broke her arm.

I was riding Chester around the sand school, galloping him around, letting him work off some steam, when a few more horses decided to join. Admittedly, I was encouraging him to go faster and faster, but every time another horse went past him, he didn't like it and began bucking and rearing all over the place. With each passer-by, the bucks got bigger, the rears higher, until the next thing I knew I had landed on the ground, head first, slamming the whole right side of my body into the sand. I landed with an almighty thud; my head had broken the fall. I was knocked out for a split second. As soon as I realised what had happened, I got up immediately, remembering my training all those years ago to 'get straight up' should I fall.

Initially after the accident I felt OK, just a bit sore. I rode Chester a couple more times after that but the last time absolutely terrified me and I haven't ridden since. I had taken Chester out on a hack. He was so pent up with energy, he was walking sideways into traffic and felt like he was about to bolt at any given time. Halfway back to the yard, my right leg went completely dead; I was staying on the horse using only one side of my body. I had always been a confident rider and spent many years competing, falling off, getting back on, but this truly terrified me. Being out on my own and losing control of one side of my body with a horse feeling like a can of pop about to explode, I felt totally vulnerable. I said a few prayers to the universe and somehow made it back safely to the yard. I looked up to the sky and said a little 'thank you'.

Only a couple of weeks later I was at home reaching for something in my wardrobe and all of a sudden, a sharp, agonising pain shot down my right leg. I could barely walk. I had pins and needles tingling all along the sole of my right foot.

After resting for a couple of days, the pain subsided and I started to feel OK again. But a few weeks later, after returning from my weekly food shop, my lower back jarred and completely went. The pain was excruciating. I tried to grab hold of the kitchen counter to support myself, but it made the pain even worse. I was confused and scared. I had no idea what was happening to my body.

I resorted to crawling around my apartment on my hands and knees. In my panicked state, I managed to find an emergency chiropractor who gave me some guidance over the phone and then came to my home and cracked my back into place. Walking to the doctors was not an option due to the pain levels and, even so, it was quite clear that the issue was back related and required a specialist.

'You need to lie flat on your back for the next two weeks,' he said.

'Two weeks just lying on my back?!'

'Yes,' he replied firmly.

The effects of the riding accident became clear. My body had suffered trauma and nerve damage. I rang my mum in tears. 'Mum, I can't do this on my own! I need you here!'

I had to resort to weeing in the shower and could barely dress myself. The chiropractor had given me strict instructions not to lean forwards so I had to keep my back straight at all times.

Mum came to stay with me for a few days. She fed me, dressed me, cooked for me, cleaned for me, emptied my bins for me, helped me to appointments and massaged my feet. That was love. Yet again, when I really needed her she dropped everything for me without even questioning it. I was totally vulnerable and living like a child again. Her stay bonded us. After the trauma of Mr M, we were able to start reconnecting again.

Things got a little heated between us one day and I burst into tears. It was all getting too much – grieving over Mr M and the pain from my back injury. Mum came straight over to me and gave me a big hug, stroking my back. 'He treated you terribly, I know it's been really hard.' Her acknowledgement of my pain meant so much. She knew that the tears were about much more than just my back and a morning squabble. In that moment, I had all the love I needed.

After Mum left, Freddie came to stay. He cooked for me, dressed me, cleaned for me. I could take my knickers off but not put them back on. So, after washing and drying myself as much as I could, Freddie would pat my legs dry and put my knickers back on, looking straight up at me. 'I'm not looking, I'm not looking,' he'd say.

I laughed. 'It's fine, Freddie, I really don't care.'

Freddie showed me so much care and nurture in my most vulnerable state. That too was love.

I began a series of appointments with osteopaths, physios and chiropractors. To this day, I still don't have feeling back in my big toe, and my right leg has not been the same since.

As soon as I was able to get out and walk again, I began walking a couple of dogs through BorrowMyDoggy. Two gorgeous cocker spaniels became my solace during the remainder of the final lockdown. It killed me not having a dog of my own but without having a garden, it just didn't feel right. So BorrowMyDoggy was the next best thing. The spaniels brought a lot of happiness back into my life as I began moving on from Mr M and once again embraced life as a singleton.

My back conking out on me was a big wake-up call. It was a reminder that I couldn't work as a sex worker forever. My riding injury was just the motivation that I needed to start thinking about retirement from the sex industry and investing my finances. I decided that investing my money so that I could ultimately have financial freedom and allow more time for family, friends, travel and helping others would become my primary focus.

• • •

As the world around me slowly regained some sort of normality, my life did not. I had repeatedly told Mr M to leave me alone and blocked him from contacting me in any way I could think of. But he continued to send me lingerie, fragrances and cards through the post. What was I meant to do with all this stuff? I didn't want it in my house. I couldn't make it stop. I did go to the police and report him for harassment but they said they couldn't take any action. And then there were the calls from unknown numbers. I ignored them, though always wondering if it was him or not. Then one day I answered one. It was one of the worst decisions I ever made.

He begged me to hear him out. He sounded so lost, so desolate, that I did. He was in intensive therapy now, he said. He was broken and he was trying to address some of the issues that he believed were behind his behaviour. He knew that we couldn't be in a relationship just now, but could we be in contact, could he show me how he was trying to become more stable and consistent in his behaviour?

It's probably obvious that I should have said no. That I should have made it clear that no good could come of us being in touch and wished him well – and blocked that number too. I did not do this. Whether by accident or because he knew exactly how to play me, he had got my Achilles heel. As an adopted child, who could viscerally remember what it was like to feel rejected and alone, I couldn't bear to hear that kind of pain in the voice of someone I had loved. I agreed to see him.

At first it felt OK. We took things very slowly and worked on a friendship, which was strange after being so intimate, but it made the most sense given everything that had happened. Still, he was trying his best to convince me that he was going through divorce proceedings and backing up his words with the relevant documentation. I took it with a pinch of salt. We'd meet for lunch or dinner, go for walks in the park, cook together, talk at length about life. Some days were a breeze and other days were challenging and emotional. Even so, it felt like we were slowly beginning to bond again.

Then, one morning, I was walking in Hyde Park and this message came through:

Dear Lizzie,

    It was good to see you yesterday afternoon.

    I am not able to give you what you seek, our journeys lie on different paths now. I genuinely wish you well and know you will find what you are

looking for and deserve. I shall not contact you again and respectfully ask you not to contact me.
    Mr M

'Not able to give you what you seek.' Um, what? I hadn't been seeking anything. I had moved on and started to feel happy again. He was the one who had wormed his way back into my life, claiming to be sad and vulnerable. Confused, I tried calling. Straight to answerphone. He had blocked *me* this time.

Despite the fact that he had 'ended it' and ghosted me before, I knew instinctively that I would never hear from him again. I should have been happy to be free, but he had reeled me back into the madness that I had been so close to escaping and now I felt like a rug had been yanked out from beneath me. I was so confused. I couldn't believe that this was happening yet again.

I began to feel total rage at myself that I had allowed him back in. I had moved on from Mr M, begun to feel happiness again, and then I made one stupid decision to take a call from a number I didn't know. He could have just left me to be happy and move on, but no. He had to take one final swipe in order to make himself feel good. Was he getting off on the power? He couldn't allow me to end it with him. He used my empathy and compassion against me to get the opportunity to be the one to leave me.

I felt utterly defeated after allowing a client to relentlessly pursue me. For me, that was the real danger as a sex worker. Matters of the heart. I had become emotionally intimate with the wrong person and it almost destroyed me.

The only thing I could do that day was stock up on sleeping pills and sob uncontrollably on my couch, screaming hysterically into my pillow. The emotional pain felt unbearable, totally overwhelming. I just wanted to knock myself out with pills. To numb the pain. Anything to stop me from feeling what I was feeling. I just did not want to wake up the next day.

ELIZABETH G.

The days went by. It didn't get better. I couldn't sleep, I couldn't get out of bed. I was in hell. All I could do was lie in my bed, in the prison of depression, staring into space. I was lost and angry with myself. If only I had listened to my instincts eighteen months ago. I feared I would never learn the lesson. My need to feel a deep connection with another human was too strong and I let myself become swept up in that feeling every single time.

One morning I woke up at 3 a.m. in a panic. My head was all over the place and I couldn't sleep. I felt totally and utterly lost. I was overwhelmed and exhausted. I was drinking to numb the pain, sometimes neat vodka at breakfast time. More than once I had contemplated suicide. I had even written a note to my family explaining that I couldn't go on. I turned on my laptop and started searching online for trauma therapists.

Looking back, that horrendous time – feeling so lost, alone – was the turning point. I reached rock bottom and I was going to have to claw my way out. It was almost the end of me but, though I didn't know it at the time, it was actually the beginning of me.

The first good thing to come from that moment of darkness was Lilyanne, the most understanding, compassionate and effective therapist I have ever met. When I was at my lowest, she said to me, 'This is just a moment.' Those words were so powerful in a time of sheer agony. It will pass. This is not forever. Words that I remind myself of even to this day when going through challenging times.

Everything happens for a reason. Mr M was the cause of some of the worst moments I have ever endured. But I have grown so much from the person I was then. I feel now that, in a messed-up way, that 'relationship' had to happen in order for things to get so bad that I finally said 'no more' and began to focus on turning my life around. Somehow I had to dig deeper than ever before, find my resilience, gain financial independence and get myself firmly back on my feet. Which is exactly what I did.

CHAPTER ELEVEN
BOUNDARIES

Once my back began to heal and I slowly got my strength back, I started looking into other options for work. I decided to return to the corporate world and got a job at a property company. I felt like I needed to be in an office around other people instead of working solo. How wrong I was. I liked the work itself, but the office was hell and only made my depression worse. I was sexually harassed, surrounded by misogynists with male egos flying around the room. My manager would shout and become abusive during meetings. He had people in tears.

One day I arrived at my desk, the first in the office, and a wave of energy came over me. I got up and left. I drove straight back home and never returned. Being back in the corporate world had only served to confirm why I had left in the first place. It did not feel natural to me to be chained to a desk, working for someone else, adding to their wealth. And while I did seem to have a knack for renting out properties, it just wasn't for me. I wanted to be building my own business.

So, after my brief stint working in property, I once again found myself struggling financially. The government-funded self- employment grants during Covid had finished, my rent went back up and inevitably I started to fall behind. I was on the verge of leaving London. I had physically, mentally and emotionally checked out and was financially ruined. I deleted my profile at the independent site and was no longer working for an agency; I was just seeing a few regulars. Again, I dug deep and found an inner strength that I didn't know I had. I persevered and stayed in London. It became an absolute defining moment and major turning point in my life.

Through weekly therapy sessions with Lilyanne I realised that it was crucial for me to start putting healthy boundaries in place with friends, family, clients, colleagues, everyone. It felt like life or death. Mr M was a prime example of what could happen when there were no boundaries in place, when behaviours were inconsistent and unstable, and I had no standards for the way I allowed people to treat me. I was proud of my kind nature, of my ability to see the good in people, but I could no longer let people trample all over me. I was never ever going to let that happen again. It wasn't worth losing my life over.

I have so much to be thankful for because of Lilyanne. She helped me to focus on my inner child and on nurturing myself. After Mr M, I realised that I just needed to 'disappear' and work on myself and that's exactly what I did. I disappeared and hustled. When I finally got my strength back and could see more clearly, all my focus was on getting on that property ladder, no matter what. I used the anger I felt at myself for letting that man into my life as fuel, as a catalyst for real change, for financial freedom and independence. I started to believe in myself like never before.

A year on from Mr M, I decided to go on a Tinder date. He was a smooth-talking Italian man who said he was 'separated'. About an hour into the date, he kept going on and on and on about how he loved how 'open' and 'free' English women were. *Oh God, I know where this is going. How the hell am I in this situation again? Is the universe testing me?* I thought. I got drunk, had sex with him, then blocked him the next day. After that I totally shut my heart off from the possibility of love. I decided I could not fall in love again until I had left the sex industry for good and gained financial independence. I truly, deeply meant it this time with every ounce of my being. Even if it meant making sacrifices along the way and being single for many years, then so be it. I was a protective mumma bear over my inner child. Nobody was ever going to hurt 'little Elizabeth' or financially ruin her ever again.

I was beginning to get a real sense of not being so desperate to rush into a relationship. I was beginning to learn to really sit with myself and my emotions. I felt a lot less desperate to be loved and was learning to care for and nurture myself. It was quite a realisation. I never saw myself as someone who was desperate to be loved and to feel love. But looking back, I absolutely was, hence going into car-crash relationship after car-crash relationship. Those relationships were never really based on a solid friendship-and- respect kind of love, but more the passionate and exciting side to love. Inconsistent, crazy love. Starting off as a fantasy but soon turning into a nightmare kind of love.

So, with financial independence in mind, I once again bit the bullet. I called Archie. It had been a couple of years since I'd left the agency. We spoke on the phone and it was as if no time had passed. He welcomed me back and I felt a huge sense of relief. I made my boundaries clear from the moment we spoke: 'My fees need to increase, Archie, I have more than earned that. No party bookings, no pornstar experiences. Clean, respectful, sensual clients only.'

'OK, darling.' He understood. He always did.

The day I started back at Archie's was day one of going over my overdraft. I went from having nothing and being on the verge of leaving London to having thousands of pounds within days. I ran straight to the bank to pay my money in. Once again, sex work had saved me from financial ruin. I returned with more drive, determination, focus and energy than I had ever had. I had a constant bullseye directly in front of me. I was not taking my eye off that target. Not for one second. All my focus was on getting on that property ladder. I would stop at nothing until I achieved my goal. I would use my lessons learnt from toxic relationships to start setting myself up with financial independence and freedom. I had a new-found confidence thanks to Lilyanne and set very clear boundaries with new clients. I wasn't afraid to lay down the law with my dos and don'ts. I began making it crystal clear that I was a sensual girlfriend experience, not a pornstar experience, nor was I into anything aggressive or degrading. I made sure they locked eyes with me and fully understood what I was saying to them, then I'd say, 'Are you OK with that?' in the most warming, welcoming way possible, but still making sure that we were on the same page. I was unapologetic to others, especially to clients, about my new sense of self. I wanted bookings to feel as natural and sensual as possible.

I moved into a new shiny apartment, a fresh start. I took a lot of pride in keeping it clean and tidy. Anyone who entered my home (friends, family, clients) were to remove their shoes upon arrival – a rule that I have always fully respected when going into other people's homes. The no-shoe rule became a test for new clients. The vast majority liked it and the fact that I was so clean and tidy because it meant that they were in a comfortable environment where they could relax. It set a tone. (I've heard a few horror stories from clients over the years about arriving at apartments to find a total mess and mattresses on the floor.) Only very rarely would a client have an issue with it. These were usually the type of clients who had an issue with getting in the shower at the beginning of the booking. I soon realised that if anyone had a problem with removing their shoes it was a red flag, not to be ignored. It usually meant that they had a general disrespect for women and were control freaks.

This time in my life marked the point at which I started to take my work seriously. It was not just a means to live a hedonistic, party lifestyle – I was past all that now. I still saw it as a means to an end in the sense that I wanted to increase my earnings and use that as a platform to achieve other things. But I accepted that this was my job and I was going to be professional about it. What really helped with this was unpacking my underlying shame about it in therapy. I was no longer going to apologise for what I did, to anyone else or in my own head. I began embracing myself fully, as a sex worker, loud and proud.

I would start any booking with new clients (and sometimes returning clients too) by giving them a 'mini consultation', as you would expect at the hairdresser or in other areas of the service industry. I'd ask them if there was anything specific that they wanted to explore or if they were more of a 'go with the flow' and 'let things happen in the moment' kind of person. I always made sure to create a comfortable and safe space where clients felt that they could share their innermost desires with me without feeling judged. I had dealt with my own fair share of judgement; I did not want them to ever feel that way. I made it clear that I was not into anything aggressive or degrading and, so long as we were on the same page in terms of sensuality, then that was usually a good sign that we'd get on well. Requests varied from slow and sensual massage to specific roleplays and dominating them with my strap-on.

Once I was satisfied with the consultation, I'd then ask them to 'sort the formalities', i.e. payment, before showing them to the shower. I never let them go into the shower without paying me first. When they were in the shower, I'd double check the money, then put it in my hiding place and start the booking. As always, clients getting in the shower upon arrival was non-negotiable. My years of experience had given me the confidence to make this crystal clear so they fully understood that if they did not get in the shower, there would be no booking. I've banned clients who have lied about being in the shower (it's only happened once or twice; I know when my shower has been turned on and when it hasn't). To me, a lack of personal hygiene was, and still is, a big red flag. Nobody likes a smelly ballsack or stinky armpits.

I was growing more in confidence, becoming more dominant and assertive than ever before. I was really owning who I was. My mind became clearer than ever before about the type of clients that I wanted to attract: clean, respectful, sensual, professional, well groomed, fun. I was not settling for anything less. I began reading more and more books. Reading empowered me: *Spiritual Economics* by Eric Butterworth, *Screw It, Let's Do It* by Richard Branson, *The Secret to Attracting Money* by Joe Vitale, *The Magic of Believing* by Claude M. Bristol and *Think and Grow Rich* by Napoleon Hill. The more I read, the more inspired I felt. I soon came to realise that the most successful entrepreneurs face huge challenges along the way. I began to understand the importance of persistence; never giving up no matter what. Of working with belief, with a clear plan and taking inspired action.

I began to meditate on a daily basis, which gave me amazing clarity and focus. *Think and Grow Rich* was the book that really changed my life. It led me to getting off the booze and drugs, which then led me to my business mentor and a ripple effect of positive changes. The flow of positivity after making just one good decision astounded me. It was a period of significant growth for me. I wasn't the needy little girl anymore, desperate to please people. I was confident, boundaried, sober, focused. I had found a genuine love for myself. My first few months back at Archie's were some of the happiest times of my life. It was helping me move on from the nightmare that was Mr M and once again my finances were beginning to build.

The final straw with combining alcohol and sex for me came via an experience with an old 'friend' from back home. Or rather, someone who I thought was a friend but, in the end, used me to get through his divorce. To be clear, I take full responsibility for myself. Nobody forced me to have sex with him; it was consensual.

He came to stay at mine for a couple of nights. I set up the sofa bed for him, not for one minute thinking that we'd be sharing my bed. The first night when we went to bed: 'Lizzie, I need a cuddle, can I come into bed with you?' I felt sorry for him going through his hellish divorce, so I let him worm his way into my bed. We had shared a bed platonically as friends before. Nothing happened that night, but the next night we went out. England were playing Germany in the Euros, London was buzzing. We watched the game at my local pub. It was one of the most exciting games I'd ever seen. To win against such old-time rivals gave the country a much-needed boost after years of lockdowns and restrictions. It was the first major sporting event since Covid and one I shall never forget, especially dancing and hugging total strangers in the street after the game.

We ended up in Sexy Fish drinking cocktails, champagne, Patrón XO Cafe tequila. I don't remember leaving. The next day I woke up to, 'Lizzie, we had sex!' I rolled over to see a used condom on the floor. It took the two of us to tango; we were both responsible. But in the aftermath, I could not help but feel anger and disappointment at myself. I began to draw the conclusion that alcohol just made me too vulnerable and people took advantage. I wasn't surprised when it was random strangers, but someone who was supposedly a friend – I didn't expect it from him. Soon after, he got into a relationship and lost interest in our friendship. To me, that wasn't a friend. That was the last drunken sex I ever had.

I became bold in my willingness to explore and started going to sex parties with a regular client that I hadn't seen in years. It was a first for us both and we were excited to venture into this world together. It was in a sleepy village out in the sticks. Only a few weeks beforehand I had been talking to a friend about all the stuff I had done over the years, and yet I had never been to a sex party. Then the booking popped up. I was ecstatic and hugely intrigued! The theme was Halloween, so I went dressed in my trusty black knee-length leather pencil skirt, black stilettos, sheer red top, red Honey Birdette bra and red devil horns. I had my bag packed with all the essentials, like condoms, lube and wipes.

When we pulled up to the five-bedroom home, we saw a hearse parked outside. There was silly string and Halloween decorations everywhere. A very friendly lady dressed in full Halloween costume greeted us at the front door. We walked into the kitchen to see a full spread: sausage rolls, sandwiches, cupcakes. A DJ booth had been set up in the lounge and all the furniture pushed to the side, reminiscent of school discos. There was something quite endearing and fun about it. Outside was a large garden complete with a swimming pool built inside a greenhouse, fully heated and steaming away. It was clear that downstairs was for socialising and upstairs was for kinky fun.

The client was keen to explore upstairs so up we went. It was early on in the evening so we expected everyone to still be downstairs. We had a look in each of the bedrooms, room by room – some large rooms, some small rooms. We walked past one room that had the lights turned off, but I was sure that I saw two faces. As it was a Halloween theme, I initially assumed they were Halloween decorations. But it soon became apparent that it was a couple sitting side by side, waiting for their first encounter of the evening. I couldn't believe it. They were just sitting next to each other in the dark, saying nothing.

They followed straight behind us into the other bedroom. They did not hold back; the woman was all over me. They were a married couple and had been to this party many times before.

They became our guides for the evening. They showed us into the middle bedroom. They explained to us that the general rule with that particular room was that if the door was closed then no one else was to come in. The husband began kissing me and my client began kissing the wife. Before we knew it, the wife and I were lying on the bed side by side as her husband began to enter me. It excited her. My client did the same to her. It excited me.

'Is she tight, is she nice and tight?' the wife said to her husband as she took great pleasure in watching him fuck me.

'Yes, she is very tight,' he said.

Suddenly, I saw light peeping through the door as it began to open. Before we knew it, spectator after spectator began to fill the room. And with that the couple we were having fun with got straight up and grabbed their clothes. We followed their lead. As I left the room, I felt a hand reach out and grab my boob. I felt like the star of the show, all eyes on me, but not necessarily in a good way. We put our clothes back on and headed back down to the buffet. I grabbed a couple of cupcakes, and we went outside to socialise.

I loved the freedom I saw at that party. There were many couples there who clearly had been married a long time. I had total respect for them to be out and about enjoying sex together. I got chatting to one couple who must have been in their fifties or sixties. They told me that more often than not it's a social thing. Sometimes they would invite another man into their home and just end up chatting and drinking all night. It was all about chemistry for them. I got that.

I'd made it very clear to the client beforehand that, 'If anyone asks how we met, just say Tinder.' I had learnt from previous experiences not to risk putting myself in that awkward position again. Sure enough, people did ask, and we were well prepared to fire back with 'Tinder'. After getting to know more of the guests and having a bit of a dance, we ventured back upstairs. By now, the party was in full swing and a full-blown orgy with porn playing in the background was going on in the main bedroom. People of all shapes and sizes, all ages, all ethnicities, in every position imaginable. Groans and moans coming from every corner of the room. The noises turned me on. Even so, we decided to swerve that one and headed to the bedroom at the other end of the house, which felt a lot more sensual. More couples having sex just with each other surrounded by other couples having sex. The sounds that they were making made me feel incredibly aroused. I began to feel ravenous. The client and I navigated our way over to the sofa. I straddled him. He came within minutes.

A few months later, Archie messaged me asking if I'd like to do another booking at a sex party with the same client. 'Absolutely!' I jumped at the chance. Same venue, same setting, only this time we had that one night of experience under our belt.

At the party, while the client was using the toilet, I got chatting to a woman named Deborah. She had been stood up by her 'sex party partner' so I took her under my wing. 'She really likes you,' the client kept telling me. Excited about our new-found friend, we headed upstairs and gravitated towards the middle bedroom, closing the door behind us. The client watched as we began to sensually explore each other's bodies.

I slowly began to undress her, caressing her breasts and licking her nipples, running my fingertips all over her body, touching on one erogenous zone after another. As she lay on her back and opened her legs, I removed her underwear and began to slowly manoeuvre my tongue around her clitoris with persistence and patience until she began quivering all over. I began to enjoy going down on a woman, just as much as going down on a man. It was obviously a body part that I understood better than a man's penis purely because I was a woman myself. I took great pleasure in making a woman cum. I knew what buttons to push.

Then I flipped her over onto her hands and knees, caressing her beautiful bottom, which she displayed in front of me, then watched as the client began to enter her from behind. Hearing her squirm and begin to squelch, my clitoris began to throb. The door suddenly burst open and in came the spectators. I could see that it made my client uncomfortable, so we grabbed our clothes and headed back downstairs. *There goes my hard-on*. Deborah stayed. I wish we could have stayed with her. But I had to think of the client and did not want him to feel uncomfortable. So back to the buffet we went.

A few hours passed and we were growing concerned that we had not seen our new friend for some time. We went upstairs and I told the client to go and check to see if she was OK. He came running straight back, smirking. 'She's fine,' he said. I had to go and see for myself what the smirk was all about, so I went out onto the balcony and peeked through the window to see her beautiful bottom perked high up in the air being pounded from behind by the most gorgeous man with a ripped six-pack. Suddenly it became clear why Deborah had stayed in that room for hours.

I became a member of the 'Skirt Club', a group for female-only sex parties. I'm yet to go to an event, though, as tickets for parties always sell out fast and need to be booked well in advance. I saw that the gorgeous Cara Delevingne did a documentary on sex recently, *Planet Sex*, in which she talked to members from the Skirt Club. I love that these conversations about women and sex in general are being opened up. Women being slut shamed for enjoying casual sex is slowly becoming a thing of the past as the world begins to open its eyes and realise that women have sexual needs too. I love the idea of going to a sex party with just women. Nothing against men at all; I love men. But working as a sex worker for many years, with men making up the majority of my clients, makes being sexual with a woman feel like a refreshing change. I enjoy both men and women sexually. People like to put labels on things, more so on humans – I don't. For some people, it makes them more comfortable knowing that they can put people into boxes. For me, when it comes to my sexuality, there is no box or label. It chops and changes, ebbs and flows, along with my mood, age, experiences. So, sorry, label makers, for me, sexuality is all about my mood on the day.

As women, we have been programmed to neglect our own sexual needs. Perhaps this has happened as a result of a sense of guilt, shame or from the messages we have received from society about what is acceptable. Not anymore. I do feel like times are changing. Sex has been so one-sided for so long. But women's body parts have not changed. Our sexual desires have always been there. I've lost count of the number of times a client has said to me, 'I'm a man, I have needs.' In the early days I kept quiet and said nothing. But in more recent years, I've found it almost impossible to remain silent, so I gently remind them, 'Women have sexual needs, too.'

I have learnt to give clients more of a guiding hand when it comes to pleasuring me. Since eradicating the shame thanks to Lilyanne, I have given myself permission to take more enjoyment for myself, to make sex more 50/50 than one-sided, both with clients and in my personal life. The best clients are totally on board with this. It turns them on too. 'Left a bit, right a bit, up a bit, lighter, lighter, lighter still. Slower – my clitoris is extremely sensitive – just the slightest touch sends me totally crazy,' I'd advise them.

As Archie always said, 'Darling, if you don't enjoy yourself then what's the point?'

I felt some sort of responsibility as a sex worker and, in a sense, that I owed it to women everywhere to speak up more and direct clients better when it came to pleasuring me. To better educate them about female body parts. Not to call me names, not to be aggressive – that wasn't ever going to help me to achieve orgasm and I began to make that very clear.

One of my regular clients recently introduced me to Bellesa House films on Pornhub – which is porn directed by women, made by women for women. The female performers choose who they have sex with. It really shows in the quality of the films. What comes across is a genuine connection rather than an all-out, over-the-top theatrical performance that feels fake. It makes the films all the more erotic and far more believable.

So I was becoming more sexually free and open than ever before. I was more confident in myself and knowing what I liked. I became the queen of tie 'n' tease, of taking my time, just like my colleague at Erotica Massage showed me all those years ago. I felt in control. Of my body, of my mind, of my sexual encounters. I had built a nice long list of lovely regulars at Archie's over the years and I began reconnecting with clients

ELIZABETH G.

I hadn't seen for years. I was continuing to build that list, and my reputation was growing:

Met Olivia around a month ago and she was amazing. She did make me feel really relaxed and after showering did nothing but worship my cock. She has an incredible body, beautiful lips and gives a really good massage.

Olivia is beautiful and friendly. She will make your stay comfortable and enjoyable. We both had fun. I do recommend seeing her. She's open minded and loves what she's doing.

I was progressing from submissive to dominant. I was beginning to feel more and more comfortable being the one in charge and having the clients as my subjects doing as they were told. Unless it was a booking with Antonio, of course. Why change something that worked so perfectly? I liked being unique and authentic in my role as a sex worker. I stopped feeling pressure by others to be a certain way. I liked to be different. More recently I have started wearing power suits and tailored trousers, to rave reviews from my regulars. I don't need my cleavage and arse hanging out to feel sexy. I feel far more sexy and empowered in knowing who I am, knowing my own sense of style and knowing what really works for my body shape. Gone are the tacky little outfits. No more schoolgirl, maids or nurses' outfits. I've outgrown them. I've evolved. Clients go crazy for my glasses and the secretary look. I've found a timeless skirt that moulds just perfectly around my arse. I don't ever want to get rid of it. Some of my regulars love the girl-next-door look and are happy for me to open the door in just jeans and a top. Surprisingly, a lot of them prefer this look and I love them for it. Getting requests for tight leather during a blistering heatwave didn't always get bookings off to the best start, though – the term 'read the room' sprang to mind.

• • •

A client that I used to see at Lust tracked me down and booked me through Archie's when I was new to the agency. It was such a lovely surprise as I walked through the door of his hotel room to see his smiling face. His name was Henry. I had previously made visits to his home just outside of London. We'd often start the bookings by eating, chatting and listening to music followed by dancing, then taking Mandy and having sex that connected us on a very deep level. It was only a matter of time before feelings began to develop. But it was over before it even started. It all got very complicated very quickly and I had to disconnect.

Years later, I received a booking: 'Henry', for one hour. I had seen a few Henrys over the years but had learnt not to assume the booking was with someone I had met before unless reception informed me otherwise. So I was delighted when I opened the door. It was my regular client that I'd met all those years ago at Lust, whom I connected very deeply with when I first started at Archie's and sobbed over when it all got too complicated. So much time had passed. All the chaos and hurt was long forgotten. I was in a completely different place to back then. I was three months sober and feeling the best I had ever felt.

Saying 'I don't drink' to clients was challenging at first but once I started to feel more confident with it, I began to own it and say it with pride. The good clients understood, even if some were downright judgemental. 'That's weird,' one said. But the more I started to say 'I don't drink' the more liberated I felt. It was like exercising a muscle. It took some getting used to, but once I had said it a few times, it started to become second nature. A no-brainer. I didn't care if it meant missing out on bookings. I knew I would gain so much more in the long run. For the first time in my life, my health was my number-one priority above anything else. Above making money, above friends and family. My health was at the top of the list.

The ironic thing was that I started to make more money when I started saying no to drinking and partying. Because I was starting to radiate positive energy and attract it back. Because I didn't have a desperation for money. And because I had more stamina than ever before. I was comfortable and I was grateful and made that known. I am living proof that sex work can be done without being totally 'out of it'. With the right level of nurture, self-care, professionalism and a good list of respectful, long-standing regulars, there is no reason at all why it can't be fun, safe and enjoyed through sober eyes.

So many people tried to undermine my progress, but I knew how far I'd come and how damn hard I had worked. It was my mindset that had changed. Nobody could take that away from me. I had invested in therapy, and an investment in therapy was an investment in myself. I took the time, I trusted the process and spent two years rewiring my mindset. I connected the dots back to childhood and, most importantly, I learnt to nurture myself. Gone was the vulnerable coked-up party girl I once was, and in her place stood an assertive, sober businesswoman with clear boundaries and a fresh focus. Those who were not on board with this grew apart from me. Those who supported the change, grew with me.

Henry and I sat in the lounge and began catching up. It had been so long, we had so much to talk about. However, he wasn't in a good way. He was in bits, a broken man. He'd just been through a terrible break-up and was struggling to move on, telling me that he contemplated jumping under a train on his way over to mine. I let him talk, I listened and offered him comfort, but I didn't give him my all like I used to. Henry had worked for many years as a therapist. He said to me, 'I can see your growth, I can see the change, I can see that you are centred.' He gestured straight up and down with his hand along the centre of my body. It totally surprised me that he was able to recognise this after years of us not seeing each other. It encouraged me even more to stay on the path that I was on. What a contrast to a few years ago, when I was in bits over him for messing me around. Still, I hated seeing him in pieces and so upset. He was a shadow of his former self, teary-eyed and vulnerable. Still snorting cocaine. We spent the whole hour chatting. Nothing physical or sexual, just talking, comforting and reassuring. It's almost as if the roles were reversed and I was the therapist. He later told me that after one hour with me he felt so much better. It always felt good to know that I was able to help someone in a desperate situation. But the difference now was that my boundaries were clear. I understood that there was only so much I could do to help.

However, not long after this Henry asked me if I could send him a number for a drug dealer so he could get some cocaine and Mandy. I was furious. He had seen for himself my growth and the change. He knew I was a few months in to living the sober life (the first few months were most certainly the hardest – I had constant cravings). And yet, he decided to message me asking for a number so he could get drugs? It astounded me. I just wasn't that person anymore. I wasn't a drug runner for clients. And besides, any numbers, any contact details I had with that world, had been deleted months ago. I left it a week before I responded. When I did eventually respond, I asked that he no longer contacted me and then blocked him. I provided comfort to him in the moment he needed it, but the rest was up to him. I realised that I could no longer 'save' people.

• • •

Reception messaged me about a booking: 'Marshall, dinner date, four hours. Olivia! I'm getting excited for your dinner date. Client says he's a millionaire!' I didn't pay it too much attention. Mr M had boasted about his millionaire status when we first met and I was probably blinded by it more than I'd like to admit. I was, however, excited to be taken out for dinner in Mayfair. It had been a while since my last dinner date booking and it would be good to get out and about among the crowds and have a delicious meal with a client.

However, when I got there, the client kept me waiting for an hour. I didn't think much of it, it happens. He still paid me for the hour he kept me waiting so I let it slip. I had already ordered myself a mocktail by the time he arrived. What annoyed me more was that when the waiter came over to the table to take our order, the client sarcastically mocked me – 'It's going well,' he said to the waiter in a derogatory tone, pointing to my non-alcoholic drink. That comment made me guarded. I made it very clear to him that I did not drink.

Nonetheless, that night he ended up extending the booking to an overnight. However, getting the remainder of the fee from him was like getting blood from a stone. It was not a relaxing evening. We ended up in the casino and he gave me a chip as my payment. He wasn't listening. I felt him deliberately stalling. Respectful clients know to make the payment up front even when extending. I did not appreciate being put in a position where I had to ask him repeatedly. I made it very clear that he needed to pay me cash, 'Now, or the booking ends.' So, eventually and very reluctantly, he went over to the cash machine and withdrew the necessary funds.

The next time he booked me was for lunch out in Soho. This time, not only did he keep changing the time of the booking (sometimes a red flag in itself), but he then kept me waiting a further ninety minutes at the restaurant. I waited and waited to the point where my blood was beginning to boil. I wasn't somebody's pet to sit around and wait for them. But it was more than that. It felt like a mind game, a power play. I knew these kinds of games only too well. My instinct was buzzing on high alert, telling me to get away from this man. Something just felt very off. A surge of energy came over me and I got up and left. I felt like I had a giant hand behind me, guiding me and moving me away. It was as if my guardian angel was with me that day.

But as I walked around the corner, there he was, walking straight towards me. *Shit.* By this point, I was furious. To keep me waiting for as long as he did and to arrive so cool and calm without an apology did not go down well. I demanded there and then that he pay me what he owed me and never book me again. 'This isn't my vibe. You need to book someone else,' I told him. In the middle of the crowds of Soho, I made him count out the cash he owed me.

'You want me to count it out here?' he said, looking puzzled.

'Yeah, I do,' I replied, looking him straight in the eye, making no apology. I took the money that was owed to me and left, hoping he would not follow me into the crowd. Thankfully, he did not.

I went straight to my local pub and ordered an alcohol-free beer to decompress. Whatever it was that spooked me about that client, I listened to it. I had learnt the very hard way what happened when I chose to ignore that 'off' feeling and be blinded by a client's 'millionaire' status. This time around, it did not impress me. Even the receptionist said to me afterwards, 'I don't think he's a millionaire, I think he's a fantasist.' I agreed. 'Tinder swindler' kept racing through my head. I couldn't make complete sense of it at the time but, looking back, that was definitely my instinct telling me that he wanted to con me out of my money, or worse.

I called Archie and explained the issue. I made it clear that Marshall wasn't to book me again. I expressed my concern if he were to book any of my colleagues. 'I don't feel good about him booking someone else; there is something that is really off with him. Lots of alarm bells and red flags,' I explained. Among his many extravagant boasts (owning half of Mayfair was one), Marshall also told me that he was a sniper in the army. He talked about shooting people and hearing women get raped as though he was reading from his weekly shopping list. It totally spooked me.

When I explained this to Archie, immediately and without hesitation he said, 'OK, I'm going to give him a total ban.'

'Thank you,' I said, breathing a sigh of relief. 'I feel very protective of my fellow sex workers and I just don't trust what he might be capable of.'

Whether he was a millionaire or ex-army or not, whether he had some plan to con me out of my money or not, it didn't matter. All I knew was, there was something that did not sit right with me about this person. I heard my inner voice speaking, I listened to it and acted upon it. Finally! I was learning.

Speaking of the 'off' feeling, more recently I had an epiphany about my intuition. It totally freaked me out, but in a very positive way. It made me realise that listening to my intuition is really what has kept me safe all these years. I had been called to a booking not far from my home, only a couple of streets away. The client claimed to the agency that he had seen me before and paid via PayPal. I checked through my PayPal history but could not find his name. Red flag. There was a lot of back and forth between myself and the agency over how he would pay. I didn't feel comfortable with a bank transfer (more often than not I would have to give my real name for the transaction to go through). Something was telling me no. So I told the agency cash only. It was decided that the client would pay half the cash to me and the other half would be transferred to the agency.

When I arrived, I waited outside the hotel and asked the agency to send the client down to meet me outside. When I heard the front door open, I turned to see the client and realised that he was someone I'd previously had to walk away from only a few weeks ago. In that particular instance, as I entered his hotel room, he'd proceeded to tell me that he was having dramas with an 'ex-girlfriend' who had been tracking his movements via his Uber receipts, which had been sent to her email. Something in me just went 'no'. Aside from him having bloodshot eyes and looking totally dishevelled, something was just not allowing me to stay in that room with him. If the years in the industry had taught me anything, it was that I knew intuitively the type of clients that were for me and the type that were not.

'Sorry, darling, I just don't feel comfortable staying here. I really don't want to get involved in a domestic. I've done this long enough and just know not to ignore my intuition. I'm sure there is another lady who would happily come and see you but I just don't feel comfortable here.' And that was the end of it. Or so I thought, until I saw him walk out of the hotel a few weeks later.

'I already told you no,' I said firmly.

'But that's all been sorted now,' he said, trying to convince me. But again, there was something stopping me from walking through that hotel door, so I shook my head at him and started marching in the opposite direction.

'Ah, for fuck's sake!' I could hear him swearing behind me. Thankfully he did not follow me. I got straight on the phone to the agency. I told them that something just felt off about him and that I had learnt over the years not to ignore that feeling. I explained he was already on my banned list.

The next day, I received a message from the agency. It was a picture of his face, with his phone number. 'Fake transfer!! Please send to everyone! Goes by the name of …' I just could not believe it. I was in total shock. I called the agency straight away. He'd booked another lady after me and scammed her with a fake transfer. That guiding hand, that refusal to stay or walk through the door, was all for a very good reason, even though it did not make sense at the time and reception thought I was being difficult. It totally freaked me out. At least it cleared the air between me and the receptionist. 'I'll always ask your opinion from now on,' she said.

The same goes for clients who are unable to give eye contact or acknowledge me on our first meeting. No engagement, no smile, no 'how are you?' Clients who look straight through me as though I'm an object not to be acknowledged get shown the door. This only happens very rarely, though. I can work with nerves and shyness – it's part of my job to bring the best out in people – but if someone is rude and not willing to acknowledge me from the very beginning, it's more often than not a red flag.

• • •

I went to visit one of my regulars in the Shard. As we looked down over Tower Bridge and onto the bright lights of London sparkling below us, the client put his arm around me and said, 'The world is ours, babe.' We then proceeded to rip each other's clothes off and I insisted that he fuck me from behind against the floor-to-ceiling window, so that I could look down over my beloved, beautiful London and take it all in. Floor-to-ceiling windows became my new fetish. At the Hilton Park Lane, I met a gorgeous client who was more than happy to take me from behind against the window while I looked out over Hyde Park. As he stood behind me, he whispered into my ear, 'I love a woman who knows her own body.' I was embracing every inch of myself and owning who I was.

There was more fine dining, more high-end hotels, meetings in bars, spa breaks, trips to Paris. One of the additional agencies I joined gave me the title 'Lady' Olivia on their website. It was never a request of mine, but a name they had chosen to give me. I loved it! Under my profile they added 'educated'. I loved the fact that intelligence was being recognised as a perk as well as tits and arse. It felt like a positive move.

'Wow, you really are Lady Olivia! All these rules … take off your shoes, take a shower, do this, do that …' a new client said, disapprovingly. I was becoming clearer than ever with my boundaries. Occasionally, a client would have a tantrum about it: it was usually a sign. 'Darling, you respect me and I will respect you and, as a result, we will have a good time. OK?' I said to him, locking eyes. I started to have a sinking feeling that the booking was about to go terribly wrong. But I dug my heels in and stuck with it. Somehow, we managed to work through it and ended up having a blast. The client extended and tipped me £100. That's what I loved about sex work: how it could surprise me at any given time. It was my job to connect and bring out the best in people. It certainly worked a treat with this client.

I still loved the job but I was beginning to turn my focus to new challenges. Playing the 'character' of Olivia for so many years was the best fun, but I was ready for something different. I did a lot of soul searching. I was looking for a new purpose. I looked back over my career and all the people I had helped. I knew that I wanted to continue helping others. Lilyanne had given me a new-found confidence in owning who I was and eradicating any shame I felt over my profession. I wanted to pass that on to fellow sex workers. I began to think about how I might be able to campaign for the rights of sex workers and transform the industry.

I was growing even more confident with couple bookings. I learnt to allow the woman to take charge – that set-up always seemed to work best in threesomes, especially when the clients were a genuine couple. I never wanted to make the woman feel in any way uncomfortable so, as far as I was concerned, as long as we worked within our boundaries, she was the boss. Putting on a strap-on and having sex with a woman while her partner watched was becoming second nature. I have been fortunate enough to meet some really beautiful women whom I have loved to pleasure. More recently, I was called to a booking with a couple in central London. It was the woman's first time with another woman. She just wanted her partner to watch. She was so curious about me and investigated every inch of my body. She was fascinated with my breasts. I loved being able to use my years of experience to help her feel at ease and give her the best time possible. We explored each other's bodies with so much respect and admiration while her partner took a back seat and watched. I loved that. It gave us a real chance to connect and take our time. Just before the booking ended, I told her about the Skirt Club. I hope to see her there one day.

Giving up alcohol empowered me. My energy levels went through the roof as I approached the six-month mark. It completely diminished my vulnerabilities. For the first time in my adult life, I was in control. I had a very clear vision of the direction that I wanted my life to go. Quitting both drugs and alcohol, in the end, was easy. I just didn't want to do those things anymore.

With my new-found focus, I gave it everything I had. It was now or never. I used all the shit from the past to my advantage. I hated how vulnerable alcohol made me and the stupid decisions I made when drunk. My blabbering mouth revealing all about my personal life to clients after a few drinks. I was never going to let any man take advantage of me ever again. The only way of ensuring that was to stay sober. I began to have total belief in myself. Belief that I could provide for myself the lifestyle that I had always dreamt of. I didn't need a partner for that. I was already living it. I had to remind myself of how far I'd come. I was worlds away from the life I had when I was living in a youth hostel without enough money for tampons. I just had to keep pushing, keep persisting, keep believing. While Londoners frolicked in the sunshine, drinking on bank holidays, partying at festivals, I was working, growing and daring myself to dream. I was putting together a plan and taking action. I was creating vision boards, writing, reading, learning, manifesting, visualising and exercising daily gratitude. Not to say I didn't have any fun in the sun – of course I did – but I didn't give in to the fear of missing out as soon as the sun came out. I stayed focused on my goals, stopping at nothing.

The longer I stayed sober, the more aware I was becoming of the world around me; I was particularly interested in the changes in the economy and consumer trends as a result of Covid. I started buying the weekend *Financial Times* to keep myself up to date with what was going on in the world. I'd go straight to the property section and start ripping out my dream homes and stick them on my vision board. I became more aware of the rise in demand for UK staycations. Since Covid, Brits had grown cautious of travelling abroad. I wanted to be a part of this rising trend. I was sure that investing in a property and setting it up as a holiday let would come with huge financial rewards. Approaching forty had a big impact on me – on my focus, on my health, on my goals, on my drive and on my purpose. It really was a combination of circumstances; hitting this milestone, the horrendous experience with Mr M and a back injury all had a profound effect. They were real turning points. Everything happens for a reason. As tough as the latter two were, I was able to take positives out of them. I used them as the fuel to pursue my goals with more grit and determination than ever before. My main goal was passive income.

My dodgy back was a stark reminder that there was a time limit on my profession. I was going to start investing and growing my finances no matter what. I was going to retire from the sex industry and use my life experiences to help others. I was still me to my core, I just was a better, sober, more boundaried version of myself. I was growing more and more into the assertive businesswoman that I always aspired to be. After years of being tested by adversity, the stars were finally beginning to align and I could feel myself beginning to soar. I felt unstoppable. I reminded myself: 'You have no idea what you're really capable of until you get sober.'

I didn't blab about house hunting. I focused on my plans and kept them to myself. I started looking along the Cornish coast where I'd had many happy childhood holidays, but prices were too high for my budget. I then thought about Turkey, simply because prices were so cheap for brand-new apartments, but then realised that it would have been madness buying my first property overseas. The whole point of me buying an investment property was so that I could rent it out and generate a second income, all while the value increased. I then turned my attention to Hampshire. It was my intuition that guided me there. I had never been before. I was blown away by how beautiful it was. I was smitten from the get-go. Even though I wouldn't be living there permanently, it was important that I got excited about it. I liked the fact that there were no memories there whatsoever. No memories or ghosts of Christmas past. No ex-boyfriends. A clean slate. I could go and visit, feeling fully relaxed knowing that I didn't need to worry about bumping into someone that I'd rather not.

. It was my second day of viewings. I'd put an offer in on a cute little cottage situated on the top of a hill with the most beautiful view, but the offer was declined. So, I carried on. I had a full day of viewings booked, eight in total. I drove straight from London to my first viewing. As I drove around the area, I began to fall more and more in love. One particular property that caught my eye was a one-bedroom apartment in a Grade II listed building with floor-to-ceiling windows, a beautiful large marble fireplace that was the centrepiece of the lounge, high ceilings, wooden floorboards, French balconies. It oozed character, was rich in history and was surrounded by the most exquisite Regency architecture. I had originally declined to view the apartment. My dad had advised me not to go for Grade II listed properties due to the challenges of getting permission for adjustments and refurbishments. I respected my father's opinion, especially when it came to anything practical. This was a new venture for me and I felt a bit like a fish out of water, so I took his advice as gospel. But something pulled me back. I felt a strong urge to park my dad's advice just for this one property. I was sold from the moment I walked in. It was love. I decided there and then that I was getting that apartment no matter what.

⋯

'Your offer has been accepted.'

I jumped around my kitchen dancing and singing, bouncing around, hands in the air, soaking up the moment like a lunatic losing it on the dance floor. I was going to be on the property ladder! Finally! I can't take full credit. I couldn't have done it without my parents' help in that space of time. I am eternally grateful to them. But also, credit to myself for working my arse off, building up my savings, not giving up, staying sober. That was the change. That was growth. I danced around my flat with tears of joy. I looked up to the sky feeling immense gratitude to the universe.

I called my mum straight away. 'Hi, Mum, I have some good news. The offer on the flat has been accepted!' I said excitedly.

'That's brilliant news, well done!'

The day I collected the keys was pure excitement. I had waited for that moment for so long. It still all felt so surreal. I walked into my apartment for the first time as the owner, taking it all in.

Absorbing it like a child in new surroundings. I walked around, looking at every inch of the property: the creaky wooden floorboards, the beautiful marble fireplace and the sash windows with French balconies. I still could not quite believe that it belonged to me. As I sat down, a sudden wave came over me and the first thought that came into my head was: 'There is a lot of work to do.' I suddenly felt totally overwhelmed.

What came next was a part of the process that I had totally underestimated. So much of my focus for so long had been all about getting on the property ladder that I didn't really think too much about what came next. I wanted to rent it out as a holiday let, so that I would also be able to go and stay there myself, take some time out of London and reconnect with my country roots every couple of months. But I really didn't consider the work and costs involved in setting up a property for holiday lets.

I spent the next two months driving back and forth between London and Hampshire every weekend and focused all of my energy on setting it up. That project became my baby. I poured my heart and soul into it. Blood, sweat and tears (literally!). I'd spend hours trawling through websites looking for sofas, beds, coffee tables, chairs. I became obsessed with colour schemes and themes and 'what would look good where'. I soon began to realise that being a perfectionist was not a good thing. It drove me a little crazy.

I had totally underestimated how exhausting it would be working on the Hampshire flat while continuing to work and take bookings in London. It was a real juggling act. I was a one-woman band. I lost count of how many online orders I made. Come Friday, when I had finished bookings for the week, I'd start loading all my packages into the car, running up and down my two flights of stairs, until it was full to the brim. I'd then drive the two hours to Hampshire.

As soon as I arrived, I'd begin unloading, not stopping for one minute. Running up and down two more flights of stairs, getting everything unloaded out of the car and into the apartment. I was exhausted before I even began. The piles and piles of cardboard staggered me; the apartment was beginning to feel like cardboard city. I soon found a local recycling centre and made very good use of it. I became hugely cautious of the effect the amount of driving was having on my body, and as soon as I felt any kind of soreness I would lie flat on my back, allowing it to rest. I had no time for my back to conk out on me.

The first couple of weekends, before the bed frame arrived, I slept on a mattress on the floor hoping no mice would come up through the floorboards. Mum, Dad and the dog came to help for a few days. They wanted to get involved. It meant the world to me. We spent the next few days painting and flat-packing together. Families and flat packs – now there's a group exercise in listening, cooperation and teamwork! There were a few hairy moments but we managed to get through it.

I also underestimated the costs involved in setting it up. I'd thought a couple of months and £2k would be plenty. How wrong I was! Maintenance works, plumbers, electricians, window cleaners, photographers, fire-risk assessments, PAT testing, fire alarms, heat sensors, fire safety equipment, lockboxes, Wi-Fi, TV, electrical goods. Not to mention artwork, furniture, kitchenware, bedding, linens, towels, decor, management fees and bills. It felt like a never-ending list of expenses that just kept getting longer and longer. But still, I had to keep myself grounded and remind myself of how fortunate I was to be in such a position. I continued exercising gratitude; I danced and sang my way through the flat packs. I celebrated my 'mini win' moments, usually with some kind of food. I meditated and remained grounded throughout. I knew that it would all be worth it.

That whole process was a real learning curve for me. It challenged me in many ways, but I enjoyed learning and understanding the property business from a new perspective. I breathed so much life into that flat. So much heart went into it. It felt so good to see it finally all come together. Lots of backache, drilling, hammering, endless trips to B&Q and Screwfix, retail parks, a few sleepless nights, cleaning, scrubbing, bending, lifting, cuts, bruises, burns and a couple of meltdowns … Two months later, it was finally ready.

I had chosen to work with a property manager. I would have loved to have managed it all on my own but felt it best to first try working with a management company to see how it went and take the burden off myself. The first few months did not go well. Complaint after complaint.

ELIZABETH G.

I was flabbergasted by the things that guests complained about. One couple refused to stay because the communal staircase needed a vacuum. Admittedly, it did not look great but to refuse to stay in the property at all dumbfounded me.

At the same time, I was not getting the bookings that I had hoped for. I assumed that because it was winter, it wouldn't be busy. However, after speaking with other property management companies, I soon discovered that they'd all been having a very lucrative winter season. My current management company were calling me with any little problem. I had hoped the eye-wateringly high management fee that I was paying them would mean minimal contact. I was beginning to understand just how much energy and work was required when running a holiday let. *Thank God I'm not drinking or doing drugs*, I thought. There was no way I'd be able to cope with any of it with a hangover or comedown. It was like a needy child requiring all my focus and attention. It was my baby, after all.

While watching *A Very English Scandal* on TV I discovered that peacock feathers are supposedly bad luck. I had bought peacock feathers for my holiday let. I try not to be too superstitious these days but because the property was having so many issues, so many complaints and barely any bookings, on my next visit I went straight over to the fireplace and yanked the peacock feathers out of the vase.

Something about my property management was just not sitting right. I was six months in, £15k down having spent every last penny I had on setting it up, and with few bookings rolling in. I knew something had to change. It was a beautiful property in a beautiful part of Hampshire. I was getting bad vibes from my management. We were coming into the summer months. My gut was telling me to start looking for a new property manager. There it was again, that 'off' feeling. It was either that or give up; it didn't feel like it was worth any of the stress considering the amount I was earning from it. If anything, I was working more days with sex work, not less like I had hoped. I had thrown every last penny I had at the property but it wasn't paying off. I took a deep breath and meditated. I accepted that the challenges were part of the process rather than letting them get the better of me. For me, that is the key to surviving in any business. Accept the challenges, embrace them and learn from them.

My new management advised that the company I had been with previously was such a big nationwide enterprise that they were not hugely concerned if a property stood vacant for a couple of months. Suddenly it all made sense why I had been getting so few bookings. I felt a little sick but, at the same time, hugely relieved that I'd listened to my gut. Before I went live with the new management, I took one last shot at it. I drove back to Hampshire and worked for three days straight, hanging more artwork, hammering, cleaning, scrubbing, washing, ironing, vacuuming, dusting, bleaching, tweaking. I booked a photographer to take new photos (as advised by the new management; they did not think the current photos did the property justice). I spent hours setting up the breakfast table, making the bed to perfection and adding touches like dressing gowns, slippers, fluffy towels and personalised welcome trays, until I could tweak and clean no more. As though I was Mary Poppins, I packed up my bags and said to myself, 'My work here is done, there is nothing more for me to do.' And with that, I drove back to London, something of a broken woman, knowing that I had given it my all.

Within a few days of going live, I received a six-week booking! I was in the bank when the booking came through. My eyes welled up and, in that moment, I knew that I had made a positive move. Eight months after purchasing the property, having dealt with setback after setback, I finally had my second income rolling in. I was beginning to fully understand what it meant to run multiple businesses and the energy required in setting up a side project while living as a single-person household. Everything was on me. No days off. No holidays. Sacrifice. But at least my persistence was starting to pay off.

• • •

As with any business, I've had to adapt and change. The economy affects my business too. For me, 2023 was something of a perfect storm. We were living in a post-Covid era mixed with a cost-of-living crisis. Trends were changing. People were spending less and working from home more. Rail strikes meant bookings would go dead. Work became the most unpredictable it had ever been. Meanwhile, my overheads – like those of most businesses and individuals – were rocketing. The sex industry is one of the most resilient industries of them all; we adapt, evolve, move with the changes. I have no doubt that more people turned to the sex industry as the pressures of the cost-of-living crisis increased and people became fearful.

At one point, my bookings went dead. Not just for a few days – it was week after week of next to nothing. The industry was unpredictable at the best of times, but this felt different. The quiet weeks turned into quiet months, and I had to start considering other options. Higher food prices, energy bills and petrol prices were affecting all of us. For me, an increase in rent on my London flat coupled with a new heating and hot water system needed at my Hampshire property all added to the pressure. My finances were under huge strain.

I have always been grateful to my regular clients and their loyalty (and friendship) over the years, but especially so during this challenging time. While the type of clients I attracted were not likely to be too directly affected by the rising cost of living, I had to be realistic. There was a certain mood of pessimism and belt-tightening throughout the country. It was clearly having an effect.

Whatever the economic situation, though, there will always be some clients (almost always new ones) who try to haggle, who push their luck.

'Three hundred pounds? Really?' I was quizzed by a new client.

'You wouldn't haggle over your lawyer's or your dentist's fees, would you? So why try to haggle over a sex worker's fees?' I challenged him.

'Yeah, true,' the client said.

I've heard this many times now and have grown tired of it. 'Can you do thirty minutes for …' one said. 'No, darling, my fees are not to be haggled. My fees are my fees.' And clients who tried to drag out the booking as long as possible were almost as bad as the ones who tried to haggle over my fees. 'Darling, the booking has finished, you need to leave!' Sex workers, particularly those who work for an agency, understand that every minute counts. Some bookings come in at the last minute, with only thirty minutes in between each booking. That's thirty minutes for a shower, hair and make-up, changing the bedding, fresh towel, tidy up and possibly a snack. So when a client decides to sit back down and start scrolling through his phone when he is already five minutes over the time, I'm not going to be so welcoming.

After taking the current economic climate into consideration, I decided to reduce my fees. It was not something that I was hugely keen on doing when it felt like the cost of literally everything else was going up, but I needed a new tactic. It worked. Within a few hours I had two bookings come in, one after another. Bookings then began to increase just in time for the summer. I was still cautious, though, and knew only too well how the regularity of bookings could change at any given moment. It was very challenging to plan a budget when I didn't know what my income would be from one day to the next, but I learnt to adapt. I wonder how the old me, who had no clue about money, would have coped in this situation. I was grateful that I had learnt a lot since the days when financial setbacks would send me into a tailspin.

CHAPTER TWELVE
LIMITLESS

During my teen years, I adored the character of Samantha, played by the fabulous Kim Cattrall, in *Sex and the City*. I looked up to her in so many ways: she was a career woman, independent, financially stable without depending on a man, sexually expressive without apology. Because romantic relationships were not a priority in her life, it meant that she could be there for her friends when they really needed her. It's fair to say that Samantha had a huge influence on me during my teenage years and well into my twenties.

My friends are such an important part of my life, even though, over the years, I have learnt to keep my circle small. Being a sex worker has meant that I've struggled to know who to trust and who to let in. I've learnt to ensure that everyone within that circle radiates positive energy and compassion. Gemma is not the only person I have had to cut out of my life because they judged me for what I do. Sometimes that judgement has been more insidious, but I have learnt to recognise subtle put-downs for what they are and I don't tolerate them anymore. I don't get angry, I get distant. I wish that person well and I disconnect. Walking away from negativity sends a far more powerful message than getting involved in the fight. In walking away, I am showing respect and love for myself. Some call it drama. I call it boundaries.

I treasure my friends from childhood. My friends who I spent summers with by the Cornish coast and have known almost my entire life. Our annual meet-ups mean the world to me and I love the bond that we share. Charlotte was like the sister I never had growing up. We have a bond from childhood that feels unbreakable. We rode horses together, went to school together, spent summers together, chased boys together, got in trouble together. It wasn't until we were in our thirties that Charlotte was able to express to me the frustration she felt about how badly my parents handled the adoption and how I should never have gone through that. I was shocked when I first heard this. I never knew that she felt so strongly about it. All the years of dealing with it on my own and there was my dearest childhood friend who totally had my back. Charlotte's protective words filled such a huge void and had my heart beaming with love.

Maria and Pippa supported me through some of my darkest days. I have always felt grateful to Maria for opening her door to me when I was fleeing domestic violence. And to Pippa, who I met up with consistently throughout the pandemic. Those days out in Hyde Park walking and talking and drinking hot chocolate were a total lifeline when I was going through hell in my personal life. Katie, Freddie, Lara and Jessica have opened their hearts to me and accepted me for who I am without judgement. Consistently. Their support has meant the world to me. I treasure friends who have been there through the good times and bad. Friends who have not judged me based on my profession. Friends who don't just want me in their life when it's fun and convenient for them, but who are there for me when I'm struggling and have nothing to offer them. That's a true friend. I was never a fan of being friends with large groups of women. I always found it too bitchy. The friendships I have are solid and my absolute treasures. I wouldn't have it any other way.

I told my dear friend Lara about what I really did for a living just before we went into lockdown. I could see that she needed time to process it but, on the whole, she took it well.

'Love you. Keep doing you, it suits you. So proud of you xxxxxxx' She was full of encouragement.

Over time, she became curious more than anything. 'Are they ever good-looking?' she asked.

'Absolutely, they are! Some days I can't believe that they are paying me; it almost feels like it should be the other way around!'

Lara laughed. 'But what if they are not good-looking?' she asked. I understand why some people ask this question, but for me personally, I just don't look at it in that way. Some of the best sex I've had has been with people I wouldn't have looked twice at if it was only about physical appearance. For me, it was never really about how a person looked, but how a person *was*.

• • •

Female sexual expression, sexual desires and impulses are beginning to take centre stage more than ever thanks to movies and TV shows. It feels like what started with the characters in *Sex and the City* deciding that they wanted to 'have sex like men' – with all the freedom and lack of guilt that men seemed to enjoy – has evolved into questioning how women really, actually want to enjoy sex. The series *Sex/Life* on Netflix about a married woman reconnecting with an ex really got chins wagging (the shower scene, oh my!). Women's sexual desires and impulses are as varied as we are. Sometimes it is not making love. Sometimes it is. Sometimes we want slow and sensual, and sometimes we just want to be bent over the kitchen table for a lunchtime quickie.

There's a lot of work to do. Women have been so programmed over the years to associate enjoyment of sex with shame, with sleaze and with being a slut. I don't have 'sleazy' sex and therefore I don't associate sex with being sleazy. I associate sex with being sensual, gentle, passionate, connected, exhilarating. One of the greatest natural pleasures of life. I have found the UK's attitude towards sex somewhat outdated and stuffy, especially compared to our European friends who seem to be much more open when it comes to sex. For the majority of them, it seems much less taboo. I would love the UK to get to that stage of openness. Women have been conditioned so much over the years. Our sex drive has always been there, but we have been taught to hide it, to feel shame. That tide is now turning. Women's sexual needs are being recognised too.

I looked up to glamour models when I was a teenager in the 1990s. I'd now question whether they were the best role models, but the attraction for me was that they appeared to be enjoying being sexy and owning their sexuality. The 'ladette culture' of the nineties is thankfully a thing of the past. We are not 'like lads', and being uninhibited shouldn't be an exclusively male thing. Female sexuality is wonderful, complex and multifaceted.

'You don't want to be doing this in your forties,' said a client to me recently.

'Really? Why not? It's the best job in the world! I get paid to have sex for a living! Why should there be an age limit? Are you going to stop having sex in your forties?' I asked.

'No, I guess not,' replied the client.

'Exactly,' I gleefully said.

In some ways, though it's true that appear to have only women in their twenties, there is no age certain high-end agencies discrimination in the industry. There really is a market for anyone and everyone, because such is the range of human sexuality. I recently watched one of Kathy Burke's documentaries on ageing and was delighted to see her interview a lady who was a seventy-one-year-old dominatrix. The lady explained that she received £600 a month for her pension and the mortgage on her house was £900 a month. So working as a dominatrix provided some much-needed extra income. And while I am on the subject of the wonderful, brilliant Kathy Burke, she also did a documentary on sex where she interviewed a male sex worker. She asked him, 'So what do most women want, they want to be taken out for dinner and have a chat?'

The sex worker responded, 'They all want sex.' Of course they do!

Every time I watch the following scene from *Sex/Life* it gives me goosebumps. The main character, Billie, confronts her mother after years and years of living in shame:

Billie: Whenever something bad happens, I hear your voice in my head, telling me it's all my fault. I've made huge mistakes in my life.

Mother: You have made mistakes. Your sexual appetite has been a problem since you were a teenager, and now it's tanked your marriage!

Billie: No, no! My desire was never the problem in my marriage. My problem was dishonesty, and the source of that dishonesty was shame. And it was shame that you taught me.

(From *Sex/Life* season two, episode two)

If being in a long-term relationship and having children is what you have always dreamt of and you are sure that that is your path in life then great, so long as it's your decision and on your terms. The phrase 'settle down' does amuse me, though. 'When are you going to find a nice man and settle down?' It absolutely baffles me when people ask me this, especially when I look back on all the turbulent relationships I have been in over the years. I can safely say that, as a single woman, divorced, thirty-nine years old, sober, focused, happy, stable, independent, with a strong sense of self, I am feeling more 'settled' than I ever have.

To all the single ladies out there who ever doubt themselves – never, ever mould your life to conform to other people. I'm the happiest and healthiest I've been in a long time. I love my single life, my independence and my freedom. I'm not knocking long-term relationships. If you're with someone who makes you happy – fabulous! But people in relationships aren't stigmatised like singletons are. Especially happily single and child-free women in their late thirties plus. It just comes down to what works for each individual, and for me, at this stage in my life, it's being single.

At twenty-nine years old, when I was still married, I had my eggs tested. I was advised that my egg reserve levels were abnormally low for someone of my age. I was told that if I wanted to have children then I needed to start trying within the next year, otherwise it was going to be very difficult for me. I didn't cave to the pressure. I never had the urge to have children, so a small part of me thought that perhaps my low egg reserve levels was nature's way of telling me that biological motherhood was not meant for me. It isn't for everyone, and that's OK. I always felt like my nurturing skills would be used in a different way, on a bigger scale.

My upbringing very much centred around the man being the breadwinner and the woman staying at home doing housework and raising the kids. It was very traditional, although in my family, Mum did also work. That was never going to be me. I don't think my parents quite realised who they were taking on when they adopted me as a baby. I think they thought I would just marry a local farmer, start producing babies and live 'happily ever after'. Looking back over my life, finding out that I was adopted at sixteen obviously had a huge impact on me. As did my family's reluctance to speak openly and willingly about it, with compassion and nurture. The wild child in me was released out into the world and had the time of her life partying, travelling and working as a sex worker. I take full responsibility for all of it and I acknowledge the things I got wrong while regretting none of it.

I'm sure at the core of it all was dealing with the inner turmoil of being forcibly removed from my birth mother. In some ways, I wonder if, in all those years of doing drugs, of being drawn to working as a sex worker, I was in some way trying to fill a great gaping hole as a result of that separation, trying my hardest to form connections elsewhere. I was able to meet my birth mother and I have tried over the years to have a relationship with her, but for many complex reasons, it never worked out. I accepted that we cannot be a part of each other's lives and have made peace with it. She gave me life and for that I am grateful. Being forcibly removed from my birth mother is a trauma that I will never get over, but it's one that I have learnt to live with.

My parents are my parents. They have shown up consistently time and time again when it truly mattered. That is love. They had their own way of showing me love. I see that now, more clearly than ever. I am so grateful for their love and the stability they have provided over the years and for keeping me grounded. They may have struggled to express emotion and give a good nurturing cuddle but they were there when it truly mattered. Through domestic violence, through injury, through break-ups, when I was working towards major life goals. They were always present. That is family. To know that you have people in your life who will always show up for you is so important. I am truly grateful for them.

ELIZABETH G.

It took me years but I finally understand why they didn't tell me about my adoption. They were scared and trying to protect me. I was raised in a very conservative family. We didn't have open and honest conversations or share emotions. Any issues just got swept under the rug. From a very young age, I had to be the parent for myself. My parents' generation was very different to today's. Mental health was never talked about. Tough love was seen as preferable to mollycoddling your children. So from a young age, I learnt not to whine or complain and to just get on with things on my own.

During my teen years, I yearned to break free from the tight restraints of a conservative family. I had such an urge to spread my wings, explore, make mistakes, learn, figure out who I was. I needed to fly far away in order to do that. Mum always said that I was an intelligent woman. I think she hoped I'd use my intelligence to succeed in the corporate world. But that never worked out for me. I used my intelligence in other ways. To build businesses, to focus on financial independence and setting myself up for the rest of my life so that I'd never have to rely on a partner's handouts ever again. I'd say that was a pretty smart move on my part.

I have feared the impact my story will have on my family. I've worked hard to build on our relationship through all our ups and downs. I hope they take a moment to understand why. This really isn't about me, it's about helping others. I also fear the impact that not telling my story may have. Of not providing much-needed support to fellow sex workers or anyone dealing with the burden of shame. I have to go with my gut and with my visions.

In spite of everything that happened with being adopted, I honestly feel that I would have become a sex worker anyway. My sensuality, my desire to be sexually free and open and to connect on a deep level all came so naturally to me that it feels like a fundamental part of who I am. Yes, in the early years, I think I translated the attention I received, the desire I could see on the faces of men, as love. It made me feel wanted and secure. It made me feel empowered and in control of my life. But as great as a lot of my clients were (and so many have been genuinely wonderful people – I hope that has come across), I was never going to find love there. If they ever did express love, it wasn't love for me; it was love for the fantasy version of me, not the reality. They were in love (or most likely lust!) with the character of Natalie, Emilia, Lady Olivia or whichever name and character I had given myself at the time.

In spite of all the toxic relationships I've experienced, of the mistreatment at the hands of men, I still believe in love. I love the feeling of falling in love. After Mr M, I shut my heart off completely for a good two years. I began to accept the fact that I'd never be in a relationship ever again. Only recently have I been able to slowly start to open up my heart again. I understand now that I must be happy with myself first and foremost so that whoever comes into my life next enhances what I have created.

• • •

The raver of the early 2000s is still alive within in me. My love for dance music will never die. My love for losing myself on the dance floor is still a huge part of who I am. It's an amazing feeling of being lost in a moment. A feeling of love. Of togetherness. Of the music pumping through my veins, giving my body a sense of freedom. I would love to one day start going to festivals again. While I'm still early on in my sobriety journey, I don't want to put myself in such a situation until I know I can handle it without feeling the urge to totally obliterate myself. Slowly, I am getting there.

Who knows if I'll drink again. I hope not. Or maybe I'll just have a couple of drinks on my birthday and at Christmas. Or maybe I won't. That is for me to figure out, nobody else. Moderation is hard. There is a science behind why some of us can't stop at one or two. That was me all over. One led to three, three led to six, six led to smoking, which then lead to eight, eight lead to five more and the five more lead to cocaine. Before I knew it, I was up two nights running, the sun was rising and I was about to enter the comedown from hell. Suddenly the people I'd been chatting shit with all night thinking that they were my best friends would become cold and distant and I'd be left to deal with my deepest, darkest thoughts all on my own. While I wasn't an addict in the sense of having a daily dependency on drugs and alcohol, it was the desire to totally obliterate myself every few months that I needed to get a hold of. It was this cycle that was slowly destroying me. This is, of course, not the same for everyone, but I now associate alcohol with being taken advantage of, with being vulnerable.

• • •

The traumas from Shaun have never fully gone away. It is not the sort of thing that just leaves a person. They remain dormant inside the belly of my subconscious sometimes for months, sometimes for years, until a trigger brings it all rocketing back to the surface again. Masks during Covid were a trigger. I didn't want to be that difficult person or have to explain to a total stranger why masks triggered me, so I put them on until it became unbearable and before I knew it, I was right back there in Shaun's living room with his hand clamped firmly around my neck, blocking my airways.

When I look back at all the years of hard partying – twenty years or more – I cringe thinking about how vulnerable I was. Running from person to person, one toxic relationship after another, a lost little girl looking for love in all the wrong places. It took one last horrendous experience for things to finally change. The situation had to get to the point of rock bottom before it could really take a turn for the better. I had to learn those life lessons in order to grow and for things to turn around. Through every break-up, every rock bottom, it was always returning to sex work that brought me back to life. It gave me financial security, a confidence boost and much-needed stability.

I learnt to capitalise on what I was good at. For whatever reason, the universe had led me to the adult industry. It was when I stopped fighting it, stopped trying to hide it and accepted it, that things really started to change. I embraced it, found freedom with it and enjoyed it more than ever; as a result of that, I started earning more money than ever. Sometimes life has a way of figuring things out for us in ways we might not expect. The obvious route is not always the best route. The key was always getting out of my head and letting my intuition guide me to living my best life.

As I approach my fortieth birthday, I feel a sense of excitement. I've always been big on birthdays. It's a celebration of life. It's a privilege to grow old; I've never taken that for granted. I'll drag out the celebrations as long as I possibly can – to a few months or maybe even a year! I've lived through trauma after trauma. Toxic relationship after toxic relationship. Yet I'm still here, still smiling, still with a positive outlook on life. Still full of love and gratitude. I've picked myself up and built myself up time and time again, learning from my mistakes. I've worked hard to get to this point in my life. Nobody can take that away from me. I've worked with resilience, with persistence, with clarity and a very definite purpose in my life.

• • •

There is no sex worker textbook, no user manual, no school for sex workers to give us a guiding light and get the most out of the industry. In other industries, you have professional bodies, unions, mentorship schemes, networking events. The fact that it is illegal for two or more sex workers to work from the same address means we cannot even set up shared workspaces or co-ops. We are on our own.

I had to figure it all out for myself, just like plenty of sex workers are doing right now. If only I knew then what I know now. Maybe I would have saved more and been in a better financial situation sooner. Through my story, I hope to give a guiding light to many sex workers out there. As I said right at the beginning of the book, I don't have all the answers. I only have my own experiences – my mistakes and successes – and all I can hope is that by writing about them here I have given you a small insight into what I do for a living.

If you are reading this as a non-sex worker and want to learn how to support sex workers better, then the first thing you need to do is be understanding. Question yourself, your own judgement and bias. You might disagree with some of the things I have written here. But I think we can all agree that a certain level of compassion and understanding makes the world a better place in general, doesn't it? I hope that one day – soon! – we will look back in horror at the fact that sex work was once illegal (I am speaking in broader terms, thinking globally. I understand that the current legality of sex work varies from one country to the next), in the same way that we look back in horror at the fact that it was once illegal to be gay, or to vote as a woman. Real change takes strength, bravery and belief. But ultimately, changing the laws and regulations will make life safer for others.

Writing this story has meant so much to me. It became my number-one priority. I know there are many sex workers out there who will recognise so many elements of my story. Who can relate. I know there are so many of you who will feel relieved, even liberated, to hear what I have to say. Every word I have written, every sentence, has been for you. I don't want anyone to ever feel the way that I have felt. For years, I felt like I was a bad person just for doing something that felt natural to me. I know that there are others out there who feel the same. My goal from the very beginning was to allow myself to be vulnerable in order to help others. I am ready. I am prepared for whatever comes my way. I feel like I have been preparing for this moment my whole life. If I can deal with abuse from people who once claimed they loved me then I can deal with abuse from total strangers.

I've enjoyed it. I'll say it – I have LOVED working as a sex worker. I have been able to help people, connect with people, nurture people, emotionally support people, and in turn they have connected with and helped me. All while earning a very healthy income, having great sex and working to a schedule that worked for me. I paid my taxes, worked daytime hours, worked sober and was professional.

I set clear boundaries. There is nothing inherently wrong with sex work. It is the stigma, the judgemental attitudes, that push us into the shadows. There is nothing shameful in the job itself.

If you are a sex worker reading this, you do not need to feel shame or guilt. There is nothing wrong with how you have chosen to earn a living. You do not need to explain yourself to anyone. You are doing what you can to survive, thrive and get ahead in life. Look at the pay gap. Look at the cost-of-living crisis, soaring mortgage rates, sky-high interest rates, food prices, petrol prices, energy prices. It's only inevitable that so many will turn to the sex industry to get through a financially challenging time. Embrace what you do, enjoy it, stay safe, listen to your intuition, set clear boundaries and eradicate the shame!

I am here to support you. Never feel like you are on your own dealing with this situation in isolation. Stand tall, be proud. The years of sex workers hiding under a cloak of shame and being backed into a corner are over. The louder and prouder our voices become, the more we take away the power of sex traffickers, abusers, rogue clients and rogue agencies. Their days are numbered. MPs and Parliament need to start hearing us. They need to start taking sex workers more seriously, form a fresh perspective and understand that it is time for new and improved laws and regulations.

If you have read this book and you are not a sex worker then first of all, thank you for reading this with an open mind. Many of us live with shame at certain points in our life. If this is you, whoever you are, I urge you now to take steps to break through that barrier. I know it's hard to and it takes time. But it is so worth it. Shame is corrosive and it stops us living as the people we truly are. It holds us back from achieving our potential. It robs us of a life full of joy and happiness. Live your life as loud and proud as you can. Break through the barriers of shame and your life will become limitless!

EPILOGUE
NO MORE SHAME

I read an article in the *Daily Mail* recently that infuriated me. The headline read: 'The "Yacht Girls" offering sex for sale at Cannes: Behind the glitz and the glamour of the French Film Festival lies a seedy underbelly of high-class escorts charging €1,000 an hour aboard luxury vessels afloat in the Riviera'. It was that label: 'seedy underbelly'. That's the narrative that people read, and which becomes engraved in their minds: that all sex work is immoral and/or sordid in some way. And how ironic that the sex workers were working at the Cannes Film Festival, with half of Hollywood there. Hollywood has had its fair share of genuinely 'seedy underbelly' characters. Just look at Harvey Weinstein. How many years was that allowed to go on for? How many more Weinsteins are there out there who we have yet to hear about? But it's so much easier to point the finger and shame female sex workers, isn't it?

Of course I acknowledge that not everyone's experiences are the same as mine. Exploitation exists everywhere, but it is the stigma around sex work that allows it to flourish. It's the shame, the bias, the judgement, the fact that it is only partially legal and therefore forced into the shadows that causes the vast majority of the problems, not the sex workers themselves.

Sex workers have long been seen in a certain light because of our profession – that we are not stable, that we don't believe in love or monogamy, that we don't have responsibilities, that we are reckless, that we are all addicted to drugs, that we don't deserve happiness with an honest, kind person. That we deserve to be mistreated because of our job. This is the stigma that has been so long attached to the profession. But times are changing. The main thing is that we are individual and we are human. We all have our own unique problems, talents, strengths. Many sex workers are stable, motivated, sober and assertive businesspeople. And just as in all walks of life, if people are struggling, let's do our best to support them. If we are to make the working environment for sex workers better then we need to come from a place of understanding. I can't say this enough: judgement only makes sex workers more vulnerable. Listening to our stories with compassion and opening up a conversation can change all of that.

Sex work is not a job for everyone, just like being a nurse or a lawyer isn't for everyone. But those who have chosen sex work as their profession deserve, at the very least, to no longer be shamed and to work feeling safe knowing they have better protection. It takes a certain mindset, a certain resilience to become a sex worker. To be good at the job I believe that you need to be someone who looks for the positive in others and takes genuine pleasure in giving and making others happy. But also someone who has very clear boundaries. Someone who is in tune with both themselves and with others.

There have been numerous occasions when people have tried to pigeonhole me as a victim just for being a sex worker. But to that I say it is no different to working as a carer, nurse or therapist. It's the same area in my view. It's all about healing, connection and helping others. But again, it's the sex workers who are stigmatised and labelled as hapless victims, despite the fact that I've never had to do a line of cocaine or drink a glass of wine before a booking to 'get me through it'. If anything, it was the opposite. I always made sure that I was sober before the start of any booking.

Let me give you one specific example of something sex workers have to deal with.

Shortly before Christmas 2022, I had a relatively minor procedure on my face (an old piercing hole that needed stitching up). I had to keep the stitches in and a small plaster over it for two whole weeks. It didn't look great but I had to work; I was in no position to take a full two weeks off. One day, I opened the door to a smartly dressed client wearing a flat cap. As we walked up the two flights of stairs, me racing ahead with the client dragging behind, I began questioning in my mind who the client was. There had been a photo circulating warning us of a client who stole from sex workers. It was very blurry so his face was not clear but he was wearing a flat cap. Could this be him? Apparently, his signature move was to pay the sex worker cash in an envelope (not unusual at all) and when the sex worker wasn't looking, he'd switch it to an envelope full of paper. If the sex worker took the envelope with the cash and checked it, he'd note where she put it and would then steal it at the first opportunity. That plus anything else he could get his hands on. But the only thing I had to go on was that he was wearing a flat cap, which didn't seem like enough evidence.

I opened the door to my flat and he followed behind me. I asked him to remove his shoes but he kept them on and started looking around at my flat. Eyes everywhere. I then proceeded to explain to him what the plaster was on my face. He took one look and bolted out of the door. I think he thought that I had something contagious on my face and that my story was a cover. I was relieved that he left.

A few days later another photo circulated of the thief. It was him! I couldn't believe it. I messaged Archie straight away. Archie replied, 'Oh, he's been around for years.' He'd change his number time and time again and specifically book new ladies who were not so experienced in dealing with arseholes like him.

I was furious to hear this. 'Really?' I said. 'Why has he not been reported?'

The fact is, most sex workers don't want to go to the police. There it is again: shame. The shame that makes us vulnerable, that allows a petty thief to steal from us, for years, without anything being done. I mentally dared him to book me again. I would not have hesitated to poke a camera straight into his face and go straight to the police and demand that they provide better protection for us.

I later heard that a couple of other ladies had kicked him out half naked. I took great pleasure in hearing this. Ideally, we would not have to take matters into our own hands like this, though. He would have been caught a long time ago.

This is just one example, and not even that much of a serious one compared to what some sex workers face around the world. But it doesn't need to happen. We can make things better if we break down the shame around sex work. Shaun tried to shame me, Mr M tried to shame me, 'friends' tried to shame me, family tried to shame me, and society tried to shame me. But it wasn't until I found a new therapist (so much credit to Lilyanne!) and began to fight back against that age-old stigma that I was able to totally eradicate the shame.

Shame is damaging. Shame is unhealthy. Shame causes people to live dangerously and in isolation. If only society could see that a bit more clearly, then it could begin to change the narrative and move perceptions in a new direction, helping to safeguard sex workers as result. We all have our part to play – sex workers, clients, agencies, society, friends and family.

I believe that our part, as sex workers, is to teach men how to be respectful towards women. It's time for change and to stop allowing clients to treat us however they want just because they are paying. When a client complained to me that one of my colleagues at Archie's wrote on the agency's forum that she wanted a client to 'rape her' I was absolutely sickened. This is not acceptable. If that's what someone really wants to do with a client, discuss it privately. Don't speak so openly on a public forum and start sowing seeds in clients' heads about how to treat sex workers, because it's those of us who do have healthy boundaries that are left to pick up the pieces.

• • •

There are many changes that I want to see happen within the sex industry. Some may seem a little out there, but that's OK. Most new ideas that challenge an age-old system often seem a little unusual at first. What's important is that we start opening up the conversation. This is where I think we should start:

- It's time to stop treating sex workers as social outcasts.
- It's time to stop treating sex workers and clients like criminals.
- It's time to stop forcing sex workers into isolation. This only makes them more vulnerable.

- It's time for sex workers to be able to openly say what they do for a living without fear of judgement and discrimination.
- It's time to start giving sex workers the respect that they deserve.
- It's time to give sex workers more rights and better protection.
- It's time to introduce proper and sensible regulation around sex work to keep everyone safe – clients too.
- It's time to offer sex workers compassion.

I hope most of us can agree on the majority of the points above. So how do we start to make this happen in practice? I don't have all the answers, of course – no one does. But I know from my own experiences in the industry that these are the things that would make the job so much better for so many:

Decriminalisation of brothels: It is generally safer for sex workers to work around others rather than having to work alone (unless they want to). The current UK law that deems sex workers working from the same space as running a 'brothel' is putting lives at risk by forcing sex workers into isolation. In my ideal world, I would set up new, progressive, government-approved establishments for sex workers and clients alike. Places of well-being. Places where both parties can leave feeling invigorated, happy and able to walk in and out of the front door without having to hang their heads in shame.

Employment: Sex workers should be able to put their profession on their CV without being discriminated against for job opportunities. I had to lie on my CV to fill in the gaps when I had worked as a sex worker. But I learnt so many valuable skills as a sex worker that benefited numerous employers. Listening skills, intuition, resilience, accounting, professionalism and organisation, to name a few.

Housing: Sex workers should be able to openly state their profession to estate agents without being discriminated against when renting or purchasing a property. I faced numerous challenges in finding somewhere to live. I had to lie to estate agents about my employment history. I felt crippling anxiety at the thought of a complete stranger going through my bank statements and asking questions.

Loans and credit cards: Similarly, sex workers should be able to openly state their profession when applying for loans, credit cards, etc., without being discriminated against.

Tax: Sex workers should be able to openly state their profession on their self-assessment without being discriminated against (ironic as it was the 'broken' system of HMRC that lead me to return to sex work in order to pay my tax bill). I know I am not the only self-employed person who struggles to pay their bill in January, after an expensive Christmas period. Personally, I think that paying taxes more regularly, every three months, for example, would help to take the pressure off. My anxiety went through the roof many times before phone calls to HMRC. I understand that feeling is not exclusive to sex workers, but the stigma around the profession certainly added to it.

Finances: It would be so useful for sex workers to have access to education and support so they know how best to manage their finances and do their self-assessment. Targeted courses and information are available for people working in most other industries as far as I can see. Why not ours? Note to sex workers: once you start paying tax, you will learn to manage your finances better and in the long run have more money in your bank account due to improved organisation of funds. There will be busy periods and quieter periods. I have learnt how important it is to nest finances when times are good.

It would be so much better for everyone if there were more accountants who specialise in the sex industry. It took me a number of years to find a non-judgemental accountant.

Let's start to shift the perspective and see sex workers as business-people. In my ideal world, all sex workers will have a business mentor who takes them seriously. Professional advisors would be easily accessible to guide sex workers on how best to invest and grow their money, whether that be in property, trading, tech or art, for example.

Health: The expectation from some clients and agencies that a sex worker is happy to drink and do drugs is wrong, and this needs to be challenged more. This is yet another way in which pushing sex work into the shadows is damaging as it makes it harder to say no and speak out.

Privacy: Though I want to live in a world where sex workers don't have to hide their profession, I still believe it's up to the individual whether they want to talk about it or not. And while we are on that point, I would love there to be some sort of protection of sex workers' identities. Newspapers printing photos or people threatening to 'out' sex workers on social media or to their friends and family are all ways that people try to have power over those who are already vulnerable, potentially forcing them into risky and damaging situations.

As I have said, there are two sides to this industry, just as there are in other areas of life. My experience of sex work, which I have shared with you in these pages, has been so positive. I love my job and I know there are many women, men and trans people out there who love working in the sex industry too. But the reality is that there are also those who have been trafficked, exploited or forced into doing things they don't want to do. I can't stress enough how stigmatising and criminalising makes things easier for the people who would traffic, exploit and make money out of those who are vulnerable.

Sex workers don't want to have to lie and live in the shadows. The majority of us want to be respected, tax-paying members of society, just like anyone else. We want the same protections and legal rights that workers in any other industry would expect. We want to get on with our jobs in a safe and healthy environment. As I said right at the beginning, this industry is not going anywhere. I wonder if the people who seek to criminalise sex work further honestly think that this will work? Has making individuals ashamed and vulnerable ever improved anything?

I want to help give sex workers the platform they need to get the most out of the profession. As I said before, there is no 'school for sex workers', but perhaps there should be. I will use my story to fight for the rights of sex workers who love the profession just as much as I will fight for those who are trafficked and forced into the profession. The more I can use my own voice, as well as amplifying the voices of others within the industry, the less power is available to the traffickers. Thank you for reading my story.

International Sex Workers' Day is on 2 June. Mark it in your calendar and let's start a movement!

Continue the discussion:

@elizabethgofficial

@elizabeth_g_official

@elizabethgofcl

Or visit www.ElizabethG.London

ACKNOWLEDGEMENTS

Writing this book challenged and overwhelmed me many times over. Lots of sleepless nights and lots of soul searching. Locking myself away in my apartment for days on end while Londoners frolicked in the summer sun. I danced and sang my way through it. I laughed, I cried and I reminisced about both happy times and sad. A lot of pacing around my flat after writing a difficult chapter and dancing to Taylor Swift's 'Shake It Off', literally shaking certain chapters out of my body. I had to open up many unruly cans of worms. That tested me more than I thought it would. But the thing that kept me going was a desire for change on a very deep and personal level. I knew that I had to get my story out if I was serious about helping others. I had to make sacrifices. I had to make myself vulnerable in order to make a difference. Helping to improve the lives of sex workers and anyone dealing with shame was at the very core of this book. There is so much more to my story; this is just the beginning.

To the many people who have supported me over the years and to those who helped bring my story to life, I am forever grateful to you all:

Lilyanne: The woman who changed my life! Without you, none of this would have been possible. Words really don't do justice to how grateful I am for your guidance throughout the last couple of years of my life. Your compassion and ability to help me get to the core of myself has forever changed me for the better. Thank you for teaching me about healthy relationships, how to implement boundaries and the importance of self-nurture. Most of all, thank you for helping me through some of my darkest days. I will never forget it.

Mum and Dad: Thank you for dropping everything without question when I really needed you. For giving me stability, consistency and a loving home. I treasure my childhood memories on the farm, time spent with the horses and idyllic summers by the Cornish coast. I hope you can understand, with compassion, why I have chosen to share my story. At the core of this book is my desire to help others. To help transform the lives of a group of people who are misunderstood. To reduce the stigma and help those battling shame. I believe that this is my purpose in life, and I hope that you can support me along the way.

My brother, cousins, aunts, uncles, grandma and extended family: I am grateful to call you family. Thank you for the laughter and for the many family celebrations that we have shared.

My biological mother and father: Thank you for giving me life.

My childhood friends who I spent summers with by the Cornish coast: I am so grateful for our friendship and all the wonderful memories that we have created over the years. Summers by the coast with you gave me a real sense of belonging.

My closest friends who have stood the test of time: My little treasures. I am glowing with gratitude for you.

Lara: Thank you for allowing me to be open and share my secret with you without it affecting our friendship. You are the kindest, most beautiful soul; my kindred spirit. I am so blessed to have you in my life.

Katie: Hugely grateful for the fun times we have shared, the challenges our friendship has faced and our sisterly bond. Your energy is just infectious!

Freddie: Your love and support over the years has meant the world to me. Thank you for helping me through some of my lowest moments; when I've been a crumbling mess both mentally and physically, you were there. And for the joy, the laughter and our many food adventures. There's no better dinner date! I look forward to sharing more culinary delights with you wherever that may be.

Jessica: Thank you for being my go-to person in high school during an extremely challenging time. I cherish the memories and your support.

ELIZABETH G.

Charlotte: The 'sister I never had' growing up. I'm so grateful for our special bond, childhood memories and the memories we continue to create as adults.

Pippa: My lockdown support. Thank you for our walks and chats around Hyde Park.

Archie: For the fabulous clients.

To all my wonderful clients: Thank you for your loyalty over the years.

To all the ladies I have worked with: Thank you for the fun times and memories that will last a lifetime!

To my property manager: Thank you for your professionalism and for working hard to ensure that my property remains busy with bookings all year round.

To my landlord and his team: Thank you for your patience and helping me to keep a roof over my head during a very challenging period.

To my accountant: Thank you for working with me without judgement.

Rhys: Thank you for keeping my finances in check.

To my massage therapist: Thank you for your magical hands and for helping to bring my body back to life.

Maria and my friends from acting school: Thank you for giving me a place to stay when I was fleeing domestic violence and had nowhere else to go. I have never forgotten it.

The Metropolitan Police: Thank you for believing me, for protecting me and fighting for justice.

The National Domestic Abuse Helpline: My angels! Thank you for listening and for providing some much-needed support during a time when I felt so lost and alone.

The ladies on the survivors forum: Thank you! Our conversations truly saved me and brought me back from the brink of hell. You inspired me every day that I was on the forum. To all survivors of abusive relationships; I hope my story helps you to heal, helps you to leave, helps you to move on and thrive as the superstar that you are.

Total strangers: Ladies in the toilets by Liverpool Street station. Thank you for asking me if I was OK when I was too terrified to go back to Ilford. The total stranger in his car at Morrisons who was brave enough to stand up for me and asked Shaun to leave me alone. The two men in the Range Rover in the car park who tried to intervene.

Big Yellow Storage: Thank you for understanding the severity of my situation and for acting fast without hesitation to help me.

Katie Piper, Lesley Morgan Steiner, Amy Norman, Lundy Bancroft: Your books helped give me the strength I so desperately needed. It was reading your books that helped me to start fighting back.

Rhonda Byrne, Joe Vitale, Richard Branson, Napoleon Hill: Thank you for your business advice and education on the law of attraction. Your books changed my life!

Michelle Visage: Your book *The Diva Rules* inspired me to get sober. Thank you.

Marilyn Monroe: We both went through the system, both were fostered, both didn't know our biological fathers, and both used our sexuality to our advantage. Thank you for your intelligence, your bravery, your progressive nature and for paving the way for women everywhere during a time when women had very little respect, especially when it came to business. Thank you for fighting for us. For breaking barriers. For your integrity. For inspiring the next generation of women.

My wonderful editor, Liz Marvin: Thank you for your sensitive approach. I could not have done this without you! I will miss reminiscing about the nineties with you.

Thank you to Anthony, Jon, Doug and the team at Palamedes PR. Your support, knowledge and guiding hand has been a breath of fresh air.

Sheeraz Hasan and team: Thank you for your words of wisdom.

Andrew Mason: For your photography skills.

Zoe Rubin, my make-up artist: Thank you for the chat and for helping me to shine.

Serenity Nails: Thank you for the years of outstanding service, consistency and five-star pampering.

Katie Read of READ Media: Thank you for your guidance.

Daryl Woodhouse, business mentor: Thank you for your expertise.

To the shamers: Thank you for giving me the motivation that I needed.

To those of you who have joined my social media and are keeping the conversation going in whichever way you can: Thank you!

To you, the reader: Sending you love and gratitude.

REFERENCES

1 'How masturbation boosts your immune system', *Big Think* (1 March 2022) https://bigthink.com/health/health-benefits-of-masturbation/#:~:text= Sexual%20arousal%20and%20orgasm%20increase,function%20at%20a%20 higher%20level, accessed: 27 September 2023

2 'The Future of Sex Work in the UK: Changing the Law to Protect Sex Workers & Providing Economic Support', *Public Policy Exchange* (4 May 2023), https://www.publicpolicyexchange.co.uk/event.php?eventUID=NE04-PPE&ss=bk&tg=bp1#:~:text=There%20were%20believed%20to%20be,from %20violent%20and%20exploitative%20clients, accessed: 5 October 2023

3 'Most sex workers have had jobs in health, education or charities – survey', *Guardian* (27 February 2015), https://www.theguardian.com/society/2015/ feb/27/most-sex-workers-jobs-health-education-charities-survey, accessed: 10 October 2023

4 'Students turn to sex work to make ends meet at university, study finds', *Guardian* (27 March 2015), https://www.theguardian.com/education/2015/ mar/27/university-students-sex-work-living-costs-tuition-fee-debts, accessed: 10 October 2023

5 'A systematic review and meta-analysis of 90 cohort studies of social isolation, loneliness and mortality', *Nature Human Behaviour* (19 June 2023), https://www.nature.com/articles/s41562-023-01617-6.epdf?sharing_ token=Q5iSjPDfWFiKc_wG2eyzoNRgN0jAjWel9jnR3ZoTv0Pp6WiL 6o0rsAZrTmzL_UN0RjM7oHAvV5vR55x3Wh_YbCWM-sDby_NFR_ tJzpil6zmEaxC4Xq5w6w3JSS8P9Fej9J-7HMagZDPwbMYoEv-W4iyq8VrK m9dSz2Q8T7kxFJ1wyT4PtDcRDg5m3jKr5sA4gFM9msFK7UUdOaLrT6 9gDImxG9VCDrM4e5ai2u7n3xw%3D&tracking_referrer=edition.cnn.com, accessed: 4 October 2023

6 'Skittles The Pretty Horsebreaker', *Historic UK*, https://www.historic-uk.com/ CultureUK/Skittles-Victorian-Courtesan-Horsebreaker/, accessed: 10 October 2023

7 'Double-life of high-end escort to fund her extravagant travels', *Mail Online* (17 August 2019), https://www.dailymail.co.uk/news/article-7366177/Sydney- stabbing-victim-Michaela-Dunn-funded-extravagant-travels-sex-worker.html, accessed: 5 October 2023

Printed in Great Britain
by Amazon